60-65 gms ≈ fat/day (handwritten)

THE "CAN HAVE" DIET AND MORE!

The Easy Guide to Informed Exercise and Food Choices

Patricia M. Stein, R.D., M.S., M.A.
and
Norma J. Winn, R.D., M.S.

Nutrition Counseling/Education Services
1904 East 123rd Street
Olathe, KS 66061

THE "CAN HAVE" DIET AND MORE!
The Easy Guide to Informed Food and Exercise Choices

A NCES™ Book

Completely revised and expanded, 1987
Revised Third Edition, 1988
Revised Fourth Edition, 1990
Revised Fifth Edition, 1992

ISBN 0-9620965-0-4

Library of Congress Card Number: 88-92532

Inquiries, orders and catalog requests* should be sent to:

NCES
Nutrition Counseling/Education Services
1904 East 123rd Street
Olathe, KS 66061

*NCES will provide free of charge their catalog which is a shop by mail
service for selected books on nutrition, exercise and eating
disorders. See order blank on the last page for ordering information.

TABLE OF CONTENTS

TABLE OF CONTENTS

INTRODUCTION

THE "CAN HAVE" DIET was first written for people who wanted to lose weight by lowering calories in their diets. It included only information about the caloric content of foods. Then, our realization that calorie controlled diets almost never work for long lasting weight loss prompted several revisions over more than twelve years of publication. In the last edition, we downplayed the use of counting calories for weight management and emphasized exercise and the Dietary Guidelines for Americans, which promote increasing fiber and carbohydrate and lowering fat in the diet.

Our old refrain "Diets don't work!" has now become more widely accepted. A recent series of articles in the *Journal of the American Dietetic Association* gave us the courage to continue our evolution away from calories as a means of weight management and toward providing a tool that anyone can use to improve their health. We felt we could no longer ignore the evidence that 90-95% of dieters fail to maintain weight loss over time. So, be prepared for our book's new non-dieting approach.

Who will benefit from using this book? Almost everybody, probably! But certainly anybody who is sick and tired of going on one diet after another only to regain all their lost weight, anybody who is interested in adopting healthy exercise and eating habits, anybody whose blood cholesterol is too high, anybody with Type II Diabetes Mellitus, or anybody who needs to lower the sodium in their diet. Does that leave anybody out?

We will be discussing more about our reasons for not writing just another diet book in Chapter One. Beyond that, our goals are to provide you with the essential information you need to bring the exercise habit into your life and lower your percent of body fat, lower fat and increase fiber in your diet, and eat according to the new USDA Dietary Guidelines. Also, we will give you tips about maintaining any changes you adopt into your lifestyle.

If your major interest in modifying your diet is to lower blood cholesterol or blood sugar and you are not worried about your weight and have not been on reducing diets before, you may wish to turn directly to the chapters which relate to those situations. The food tables are present to assist all readers in making informed choices of the food they eat.

If you have been on any diet to lose weight, please start at the beginning with Chapter One. We hope you'll be glad you did.

Chapter 1

TO DIET OR NOT TO DIET?

Many of you reading this book will be starting on yet another quest to lose weight. You have in mind the all too dismal picture of unsuccessful efforts to pare your body down to a size you believe society will find "good," only to find your weight creeping up (after a few months or years) to at least what it was before you started tinkering with it. People who go on a diet stand a better chance of winning a lottery than of keeping the weight off.

Yet we are all bombarded with the latest "Miracle Diets" which guarantee you will lose weight permanently! Even health professionals are getting in on the act with medically supervised fasts. Unfortunately, at this writing, these very expensive and sophisticated programs do not have any better track record over time than any other diets. We will be delighted to change that statement if someone can prove us wrong.

Respected professionals in the fields of weight management and eating disorders have stated that in no other medical condition is a treatment with a failure rate of 95-98% allowed to continue.

Susan Wooley, Ph.D., an expert in eating disorders, has posed the question, "If we don't have treatments that work, why should we use ineffective treatments?" For treatments that don't work, we spend an enormous amount of money, approximately $32 billion in 1990. It is estimated this figure will rise to $51 billion by 1995. When we see the ads and commercials for weight loss treatments, the people pictured in them have just finished a round of dieting and have successfully lost weight as most people do on a diet. What we don't see are the results down the road when they have regained that weight and more (and, perhaps have been on additional diets).

A recent study suggests that fluctuations in body weight are implicated in increased risks of coronary heart disease and death. Questions are being raised by experts in the field about the possible long term health hazards associated with dieting and gaining, and dieting and gaining.

We agree with the researchers who propose that all weight reducing programs should be viewed as experiments, with full disclosure that long-range results may not meet your expectations.

WHAT ARE OTHER COSTS OF DIETING?

Dieting may make you fatter! What the weight loss hustlers don't tell you is that every time you go on a low calorie diet, your calorie needs go down. This is nature's way of conserving the body during a period of starvation. This is how human beings have survived famines throughout the centuries.

Let us give you an example of what this means to a dieter. Marie, a

41 year old inactive woman who weighed 157 pounds and was 5'2" tall, had an estimated total caloric need of approximately 2000 calories per day. She began a popular low carbohydrate diet of 800 calories per day. At first, her losses were impressive, and she did reach her goal weight. However, when she came to see us, she had gained back all of her losses and 10 pounds more! She claimed she could not eat over 1400 calories per day without gaining weight. Was she lying, as many health professionals used to think when someone made that claim? Almost certainly not, since we now have seen that severely restricted diets can lower calorie needs by as much as 15-30% below pre-dieting levels. Marie's pre-diet calorie need level of 2000 per day, less 30%, equals 1400 calories—about what she claims she can eat without gaining weight.

If you have experienced the "yo-yo" effect, or as some wags call this phenomenon "The rhythm method of girth control" (repeatedly losing and regaining more than you lost), you can now understand why that may have happened. After Marie lost weight on the very low calorie diet, her calorie needs were lower than when she started dieting. When she resumed more normal eating habits, she gained weight. We have known for many years that the body's response to starvation is to lower calorie needs in an attempt to preserve life as long as possible. The "problem" with our bodies is that they cannot tell the difference between dieting and starving.

Some studies have shown that with each attempt at dieting, weight loss becomes progressively slower and weight gained after dieting comes back faster.

YES, BUT I HAVE HEARD OF RECENT STUDIES WHICH SAY CALORIE NEEDS ARE NOT LOWERED WITH DIETING.

We've heard the same reports and after reading the original articles these reports were based on, we are staying with the previous studies which show that dieting lowers calorie needs. The fact is most respected authorities believe that a decrease in calorie needs is a result of a decrease in lean body mass (mostly muscle and bone) due to aging, lack of exercise and/or dieting to lose weight. Once lean body mass (LBM) is decreased, calorie needs are decreased and the body very efficiently stores any extra calories as fat.

The new reports are based on studies presented at an international conference on very low calorie diets (VLCDs). Some of the authors of these studies attempted to discount the impact of dieting on basal metabolic rate. Your basal metabolic rate is the number of calories you need just to sustain your body's vital functions while you are awake. This accounts for most of your daily calorie needs. It is interesting to note that the new reports and this conference were sponsored by companies involved in the production, distribution and sales of VLCDs to the medical doctors who use them to treat obese patients—a very lucrative business indeed.

SO IF I DO LOSE SOME LEAN BODY MASS DURING MY DIET, WHAT'S THE BIG DEAL?

When you lose some of your muscle mass, you lose some of your calorie burning machinery. It's mainly the muscles that burn calories. And keep in mind, your vital organs such as heart, kidneys, etc. are part of your LBM and could be harmed. Organ failure has been reported in people who diet to extremes. If this isn't enough to scare you off, consider what it means to women. Every time a woman diets without some form of exercise, she loses not only some muscle, but probably some bone mass as well. This loss of bone undoubtedly increases her chances of developing osteoporosis. Also, many of these heavily promoted diets forbid her from eating the best food sources of calcium such as low fat dairy products. For those of you who feel safe because you are taking calcium supplements, don't count on these for protection from bone problems later on. Some research shows that it is the food sources of calcium that may be best at preventing bone problems. Furthermore, it is your lifetime intake of calcium that appears to offer the best prevention of osteoporosis.

We are scared to death, frankly, because of more and more reports of young girls "dieting". A survey of San Francisco parochial schools turned up the alarming information that almost half of 9–year–old girls and almost 80 percent of 10 and 11–year–olds reported dieting to lose weight. Fifty–eight percent of the 500 girls studied considered themselves overweight although analysis of their height and weight showed that only 17 percent were. Children and young teenagers who diet have more to lose than weight; they put their growth and development, not to mention their self-esteem, in jeopardy.

BUT, I ALWAYS FEEL SO GOOD ABOUT MYSELF WHEN I AM ON A DIET!

That may be true as long as you are doing well and losing weight. But, how do you feel when the weight starts creeping upward again, or if you find yourself in the middle of a binge? The psychological effects of bingeing and/or not maintaining weight losses are significant. To illustrate, we remember Jenni who was a world class dieter and could peel off pounds rapidly when she was on a diet. She reported an intense "high" feeling as long as her eating was under control. As soon as she got within 10-15 pounds of her "goal" weight, she would begin out of control binge eating. She felt extreme self disgust, a sense of failure, guilty, and ashamed; she could do nothing right. In short, she was severely depressed. Does this sound familiar?

WHY DO PEOPLE ALMOST ALWAYS BINGE DURING OR RIGHT AFTER A DIET?

The debate goes on as to whether people binge for psychological or physiological reasons. It should be no surprise that a body in a state of starvation (a reducing diet) will crave food and that even well disciplined dieters will eventually succumb to this physiological need. In the 1940's, Ancel Keys, M.D., conducted a classic starvation experiment on conscientious objectors (World War II). These men were normal physically and psychologically and were placed on about one-half their normal intake of calories.

As the experiment went on, the men became obsessed with food, spent long hours planning menus and poring over cookbooks. One was found rooting through garbage cans. Several began collecting and hoarding strange items, a behavior observed in starved animals. Others found themselves bingeing out of control and felt the same self-loathing and contempt that the bingeing dieter does. Although the men were reported to have quite tolerant dispositions before the study, they be-came more anxious, felt nervous and irritable with frequent outbursts of anger. They lost interest in the opposite sex and withdrew socially. In addition to being depressed, the men were found to have impaired concentration, alertness and judgment. At least two were admitted to the psychiatric ward of the hospital. Basal metabolic rate was lowered by as much as 40%.

When refeeding began, obsession with food and its preparation continued. Several reported bingeing. Body weight rebounded, reaching 10% above original levels and body fat outdistanced original levels by 40%.

Many of the findings of this study parallel what happens to a dieter and help illustrate the exceptional resistance of normal individuals to weight loss.

In other words, overzealous dieting (below 1200 to 1400 calories or fasting) and/or excessive exercising may lead you not only to binge, but can cause a host of physiological and psychological consequences. Bingeing is one way your body has of telling you that it is starving and it is time to take a breather from overly strict efforts to lose weight.

When people persist in setting unreasonable and unrealistic weight loss goals, they almost always find themselves in a vicious cycle of too strict dieting, too much exercise, binge eating, followed by feeling guilty and hating themselves. Once they are in this cycle, they are usually doomed to repeating it over and over again. If this should happen to you, seek help from a health professional who is skilled in handling compulsive eating or binge eating problems. Continued dieting will only prolong your problem. In fact, almost all people who develop anorexia nervosa (self-starvation) and bulimia nervosa (severe binge eating and purging) have been on a diet to lose weight before the development of their eating disorder.

CYCLE OF THE TYPICAL DIETER

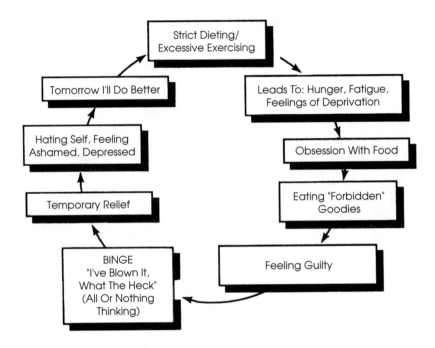

Our bias is that the binge stems from a physiological need for an adequate nutrient intake and psychological problems are secondary. This topic deserves more discussion than this small book can provide.

WHY SHOULD I CONTINUE READING THIS BOOK IF DIETING DOESN'T WORK?

As we stated in our introduction, our goal is to give you tools to help you adopt the exercise habit into your life and to help you learn to eat healthier by lowering fat and increasing fiber in your diet. These steps can lower your body fat and will result in a trimmer and healthier you. Your self-esteem **can** be improved. And you may lose pounds too! Read on to see how you can take these steps to a healthier you.

IN A NUTSHELL

1. Dieting doesn't work for long lasting weight loss.
2. Be aware of the effect of dieting on the body.
3. Be aware of the effect of dieting on your self-esteem.
4. Be aware of the cost of dieting to your pocketbook. There is a bottom line. Diet programs promising quick weight loss have gained "fat" profits from the dollars of people who eventually gain just fat.
5. Dieting can lead to serious eating disorders such as anorexia nervosa and bulimia nervosa.

Chapter 2

THE WEIGHT OF THE MATTER

Most of you reading this book are, no doubt, reading it under the assumption you still need to lose weight. In our society, what is thought to be "fat" and what is thought to be "thin" has more to do with fashions of the "in" body style than with potential medical problems. As a matter of fact, if you trace the "in" body styles, they change quite frequently. From the rounded, voluptuous female forms of the Renaissance to the flat chests of the 20's, to Marilyn Monroe's curves of the 50's, to today's athletic, no fat build, you can see the ideal body style is dictated by fashion, rather than Mother Nature. How many of us can be "in" with our shape? Look around and note the wide variety of human forms and shapes. You can quickly see that not too many are "in" at the moment. Our advice is to make the best of the shape Mother Nature gave you by exercising and eating healthy.

HOW DO I GO ABOUT BEING THE BEST I CAN BE?

The best advice is to come as close as you can to a desirable level of body fat. If your level is too high, exercise and eat less fat. But, before you do anything, find out how fat you are.

This is not as easy as looking up your weight on a chart. The standard height/weight tables are still the most commonly used methods to determine so-called "ideal" or "desirable" body weight. This is probably because they are so readily available and easy to use. After debating whether to include these tables again, we decided to omit them in the body of the text. Look in Appendix A on page 125 if you feel the urge to check out your frame size and weight range.

Do these charts tell all? In a word, no! Unfortunately, determining degree of fatness from a standard height/weight table, even when body frame size is taken into account, can be fraught with error. Body weight is composed of lean body mass and body fluid as well as fat. The weight on the scale cannot tell you the proportion of each. But **your** best weight may depend on that proportion.

Although the optimum level of fat probably varies from person to person, highly regarded exercise physiologists McCardle, Katch and Katch suggest the desirable level of body fat for men is 15 percent or less and 25 percent or less for women. Total body fat is not the whole story either—it is broken down into storage fat and what is termed "essential" fat.

For men, 3 percent body fat is essential and appears to be the rock bottom level. Below this, normal physiological functioning and capacity for exercise may be impaired. The rock bottom level of essential body fat for women to maintain good health appears to be 12 percent. It is thought that the higher level of essential fat in women has to do with their reproductive functions—that a woman needs a certain amount of fat in order to ovulate, conceive and carry a fetus to full term.

Although the minimum amount of total body fat (essential plus storage) for women is controversial, many experts have found, depending on the individual, that women who fall below 13–17 percent body fat risk stopping their menstrual periods. Some authorities consider 22 percent fat in women to be necessary for normal hormonal function. Furthermore, there is considerable evidence that female athletes or people with anorexia nervosa who drop their body fat below their optimum level may develop premature osteoporosis (loss of bone mass). More study is certainly needed in this area to protect the health of women of all ages, especially competitive athletes. We are aware of the pressure placed on these athletes to maintain quite low body fat percentages. The 1992 Olympic female athletes appeared less fat than ever, and we wonder if they are below the essential level of fat for women.

AT THE OTHER END OF THE SCALE?

What is overfat? Overfatness has been defined as above 20 percent body fat for young men and 30 percent for older men. These percentages are above 30 for overfat young women and 37 for overfat older women.

How do you determine if you are over or under fat or just right? We recommend seeking out a health professional who can help you determine your body fat percentage. The most commonly used and least expensive methods are either circumference or girth measurements of selected body sites, or skinfold measurements which assess subcutaneous (just below the skin) fat, using skin calipers. A combination of measurements from three or more body sites will give an estimate of body fat percentage with either of these methods. The accuracy of skinfold measurements depends on the skill and training of the clinician taking them. Other methods used to determine body fat percentage are less readily available and require sophisticated, expensive equipment. These include underwater weight tanks, whole body potassium counters, and electrical impedance devices, to name a few.

AM I TOO FAT?

The next table will help you determine this after you have had your body fat percentage measured.

TABLE 2–1		
	MEN	**WOMEN**
Too Low Level of Fat	**3% or Less**	**17% or Less**
Desirable Fat	15% or below	22–25%
Overfat		
Young	20% or above	30% or above
Older	30% or above	37% or above

An example of a client who came to see us for binge eating problems and to lose weight will help illustrate how knowing the percentage
of body fat can help set a more realistic goal.

Irene weighed 187 pounds and was 5'2" tall with a large frame. Irene
had been lifting weights as part of her fitness program and had a rather
stocky body build. She felt terrible about her "excess" weight because
according to the Height and Weight Tables (see Appendix A on page
125) she should weigh between 140–159 pounds.

But her body fat percentage was estimated at 27.4 percent using skin
calipers. This percent translates into 51 pounds of body fat (187 pounds
times .274). She had an estimated lean body mass (LBM) of 136 pounds
(187 minus 51 pounds of fat). At the lower end of her recommended
weight range (140 pounds), she would have been allowed to have only
about 4 pounds of body fat (140 minus 136 pounds of lean body mass).
Four pounds of fat would represent only about 3 percent body fat—well
below the essential fat level for women.

If her goal is to have a body fat percent of 25, with a lean body mass
of 136 pounds, she could weigh 181 pounds (136 pounds LBM plus 45
pounds body fat = 181 pounds).

Needless to say, Irene was relieved to know that if she achieved the
desirable level of 25 percent fat, she would not have to lose below the
175-180 pound range. For her to achieve even her highest
recommended weight on the Height/Weight chart of 159 pounds, she
would have to sacrifice some of her lean body mass. In the past, her
efforts to maintain weights below 170 pounds had met with failure because her body was fighting this loss of muscle mass. Unfortunately,
individuals with well developed muscle mass often are ill–advised by
themselves and others when they attempt to achieve these unrealistic
weight goals.

If we saw Irene today for the first time, we would not be discussing
weight goals with her, but instead would figure her lean body mass and
her body fat percent. Then, we would work with her on refining her
exercise program and on healthy eating.

Binge eating is not an uncommon symptom in this situation. Irene's
too rigorous, low carbohydrate, low calorie dieting efforts, coupled with
her exercise program, led to frustration, guilt, and anxiety from repeated
"compulsive" overeating (binge eating). When Irene adopted a diet with
more carbohydrate, less fat, and more calories, her body ceased to fight
back. Her binge eating stopped and her weight began to slowly decrease. Now you can see why we strongly urge you to seek out a professional who can assess your body fat percentage and help you set
reasonable, realistic goals before you undertake a weight loss program.
Otherwise, you may find yourself joining the legions of unhappy dieters
who are striving to achieve the impossible and end up caught in the
vicious cycle of dieting and bingeing.

IN A NUTSHELL

1. Don't let fashion dictate your shape.
2. Find someone who can determine your body composition before undertaking your "best I can be" program.

Chapter 3

USE 'EM OR LOSE 'EM

One of the purposes of this book is to provide the reader with assistance in choosing appropriate exercise for physical fitness and lowering body fat. There are many in depth physical exercise books which we recommend on pages 134 and 135. However, our purpose in the next few chapters is to provide you with a starter kit because we think several key points need to be made with regard to exercise, fitness and body fat management.

The old adage, "Use' em or lose 'em," certainly applies here. As we grow older and/or exercise becomes more of a spectator sport, what happens? We get a well-padded seat and well marbled muscles throughout our body. Muscle cells that are unused grow smaller while the fat cells are growing larger. When we start to move our legs and arms again, the muscle cells increase in size and fat cell size decreases. The result is an increase in our basal metabolism, not the decrease that you will get if you diet without exercising.

CAUTION! Some studies have shown that even though a person engages in exercise, if he/she goes on a very low calorie diet, metabolic rate drops anyway.

It appears that the best way to lower body fat is to engage in some form of aerobic activity. Aerobic means air and specifically the oxygen in the air. Any exercise which moves the large muscle groups (arms and legs) consistently over a period of time increases the muscles' use of oxygen and is therefore considered aerobic. Aerobic exercise also results in a slight increase in your resting metabolic rate for several hours after the exercise takes place. Exercise keeps you from losing that all-important lean body mass that happens if you only diet. We believe that people who need to lose fat are better off if they begin their fitness programs before they begin changing their diet. People who exercise will most likely avoid the post-dieting increase in weight we discussed earlier.

WHAT EXERCISE DO YOU CHOOSE?
Before you choose anything, see your physician and get a green light.

We can tell you that several studies have shown that walking, bicycling, and running are some of the more effective ways of reducing body fat. These are all forms of aerobic exercise. Other forms include swimming, rowing, dancing, jumping rope, running in place, cross-country skiing, ice skating, roller skating, and the recently popular stair-stepping.

Most people do best if they pick an exercise they enjoy doing. We recognize that many overfat people have never had a history of doing any kind of exercise and feel a great reluctance to even think about any form of movement, strenuous or otherwise. We also know a few of you out there, ourselves included, who say, "But, it's so bo-or-ring!" Our advice to the latter is to adopt the motto, **"Better bored than broad!"** After all, what is the alternative? You can stay with your sedentary habits and your fat cells will continue growing in size, and perhaps in number. The choice is yours!

MODESTY BECOMES YOU!

In this case, we are not thinking of the type of clothing you select for your exertions, but of the size of your exercise goals. For those of you who have no recent exercise history, it is important that you set very small goals in the beginning—perhaps something as modest as walking for five minutes around your house. You can build from there.

To illustrate, let's use Carolyn as an example. Carolyn had never engaged in anything more strenuous than cooking and keeping house. In her childhood, it was considered unladylike for young girls to be sports minded. When we first saw her, she professed a strong dislike for anything connected with any extra movement. She was 62 years old, 5 feet tall, and weighed 187 pounds. In addition, she had a spinal injury which left her in constant pain and on a strong pain medication.

This was Carolyn's program: Convinced of the importance of exercise in any responsible health improvement program and with her doctor's encouragement, Carolyn set, as her first goal, to walk for five minutes on her carpeted basement floor every other day for one week. The next week she moved up to seven minutes every other day. The third week saw her go to ten minutes every other day. To make a long story short, Carolyn was able to increase her walking gradually, up to a total of 45 minutes four to five times each week. And she graduated from her basement to the shopping centers. As she gained muscle strength, her back pain decreased somewhat.

PATIENCE IS A VIRTUE

It took several months before weight loss occurred for Carolyn. Her net loss over a six month period was five pounds, most of this occurring the last month. Her caloric intake ranged between 1200 to 1400 calories per day, according to her food records. Although we did not measure Carolyn's body fat, we are speculating that because Carolyn was so out of shape and had lost so much muscle tissue due to aging, previous reducing diets and inactivity, it took awhile for her to regain enough muscle mass to increase her metabolic rate.

Most people would have given up in disgust with this small weight loss. But Carolyn persevered because she was feeling so much better with her walking program. She realized that her greatest hope for losing fat was to gain muscle mass. The moral of this story is to hang in there, even when the task seems impossible. Remember Carolyn! Many others we have worked with have surmounted what seemed to be impossible odds because they made a commitment and believed they could do it.

One other point is worth mentioning before we leave this section. People who engage in weight loss programs want to lose weight and want to lose it NOW! But if you begin exercising at the start of your weight management efforts, be prepared for little or no weight loss at the beginning. What's happening is you are gaining muscle mass.

Gary's case illustrates this point. Gary arrived in our office committed to doing everything right. He kept meticulous diet and exercise records from the very start. Gary chose a walking program which he was able to implement quite easily since he was a relatively young man without any health problems. Within a few weeks, Gary was walking 45 minutes to 1 hour a day four to five days a week. He increased his carbohydrate intake and lowered his fat intake somewhat. Gary expected to see his pounds magically melting away. However, his body weight actually increased by two pounds.

Gary was distraught until we showed him how his body composition had responded to exercising. When we measured his skin folds, we calculated he had lost about seven pounds of fat and had gained about 9 pounds of muscle mass. This gain in muscle weight accounted for the 2 pound total weight gain. Even without an actual drop in pounds, his body measurements were changing to the point that he was developing "baggy pants syndrome".

The chart below will help illustrate what happened with his body composition.

GARY'S BODY COMPOSITION CHANGE			
	WEIGHT	# OF FAT	# OF LEAN
Initial	250	50	200
Later	252	43	209

As Gary exercised, his muscles "firmed up" and his body began to regain a more youthful appearance. Had he not exercised and just dieted, his weight would have dropped, but his body shape would just have been a smaller edition of its fatter self and not as youthful-appearing. He probably would have experienced a decrease in muscle mass with little or no decrease in body fat percentage.

Research has shown that in some cases it can take a minimum of two months before any weight loss shows up on the scales when you begin exercising as a part of your weight management program. If a person is older and out of shape, it may take even longer. This situation is difficult for the impatient dieter who wants immediate gratification.

Most popular weight loss schemes promise immediate results and often brag, "No exercise is necessary!" There is no question about it, they do deliver fast weight losses, but at what expense? You have been robbed in your pocketbook, and probably of your chances for perma- nent weight loss. It is well known by most health professionals that fast weight loss is composed primarily of water and lean body mass. We can certainly see why promoters of quick weight loss programs do not emphasize exercise as part of their approach. If they did give you the true facts, few would enroll in their programs because exercise usually slows down initial weight loss. Exercise speeds up fat loss but also promotes an increase in LBM which weighs heavier than fat.

A WORD TO THE WISE: IF YOU ARE SERIOUS ABOUT LOSING SOME OF YOUR BODY FAT, YOU ARE MAKING A PERMANENT COMMITMENT ONCE YOU START EXERCISING. If you stop exercising, your weight will increase, just as it does when you stop dieting. And, when you stop both dieting and exercising as many do, watch out!

IN A NUTSHELL

1. Start with modest exercise goals.
2. Be patient.
3. Know your body composition before and during your program.

Chapter 4

SAFETY FIRST

Remember our illustration using Carolyn in Chapter Three where we stressed a modest exercise goal? Instead of trying for an Olympic Gold Medal the first time around the block, you might want to shorten the event. The old exercise philosophies of "No pain, no gain" and "More is better" have lost their credibility and should be buried along with all your old diets. Current exercise practices stress "The FITT Principle": Frequency, Intensity, Time and Type. This means you need to think about how often, how hard, and how long you need to exercise, as well as what type of exercise to choose.

How often do you need to exercise? Somewhere between three and five or six times per week, depending on whether you are simply interested in conditioning your aerobic systems or are using exercise as a fat loss aid. Aerobic exercising three or four times per week is usually recommended for increasing cardiovascular fitness. For weight loss, the long term goal is to exercise five or six times per week.

HOW HARD DO I EXERCISE?

This is an area of great concern. The typical exerciser shows up with more enthusiasm than knowledge about how to begin a fitness program. We have all probably experienced "the morning after" the day before when we overdid.

If you want to avoid "the morning after" or the pain of strain or possibly a worse fate, monitoring your pulse rate while exercising can help. Some authorities suggest skipping the pulse rate test and using the talking pace test. If you are too winded to carry on a limited conversation with someone, you are exercising at too high an intensity and may be doing yourself more harm than good. To discover whether you are exercising hard enough for an aerobic benefit, you will want to discover how to take your pulse.

Use your index finger to count your heart beats on the thumb side of your wrist or on the carotid artery in your neck just below your jaw. See the diagram below for the proper technique.

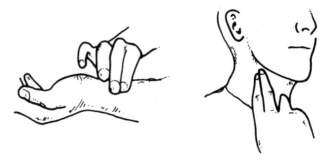

When you are just starting out, you will want to check your pulse in the middle of and perhaps several more times during your exercise session, especially if you find yourself out of breath. Practice counting your pulse for 10 second intervals until you are able to take it easily when you are not exercising. When you begin taking your pulse during exercise, continue the 10 second count and multiply by 6 to know how fast your heart is beating per minute. Training heart rate (THR) refers to the desirable range of heart beats per minute to obtain an aerobic training effect. It is important to know what your maximum heart rate is and what your training zone is.

MAXIMUM HEART RATE

Unless you have had a stress test and your doctor has told you about your maximum heart rate level, you can estimate your theoretical maximum heart rate by subtracting your age from 220. To save wear and tear on your calculator and/or brain, you can consult the chart below not only for your maximum heart rate, but also for the heart rates which will put you in your appropriate THR zone.

When you are just starting out, especially if you are older or out of shape, you will need to be at or below 65 percent of your maximum level.

TABLE 4-1
TRAINING HEART RATES

AGE	MAXIMUM HEART RATE	BEATS PER MINUTE			10-SECOND PULSE COUNT	
		LOW (65%)	HIGH (80%)	ATHLETE (85%)	LOW	HIGH
20	200	130	160	170	23	27
25	195	127	156	166	23	26
30	190	124	152	161	22	25
35	185	120	148	157	22	25
40	180	117	144	153	21	24
45	175	114	140	149	20	23
50	170	111	136	145	20	23
55	165	107	132	140	19	22
60	160	104	128	136	19	21
65	155	98	120	132	18	20

DOES THIS TABLE APPLY TO ME?

According to Covert Bailey, in his book *THE NEW FIT OR FAT*, approximately 15% of you will have slow beating hearts, 15% of you will have fast beating hearts and about 10% of you will be taking medication such as beta blockers that affect heart rate during exercise. If you are among this 40%, the table is meaningless. You will need to use the talking pace test mentioned earlier. As a matter of fact, everyone can use the talking pace test. However, for the 60% of you who have a normal heart rate response to exercise, the table can be a valuable tool to keep you from overdoing it.

DO, BUT UNDERDO! is a good phrase to keep in mind here. The higher level (85 percent of your maximum) is reserved for young people and well-trained athletes. If by chance you should find your heart beating above 80 percent of your maximum, slow down! You may be harming yourself and will probably quit your exercise program within a very short period of time.

A warming up period is essential—just start off your walk or other exercise at a very slow pace and gradually increase until you are within your THR.

Just as important is a cooling down period when you have completed the time you wish to spend in your THR zone. The cooling down period allows the blood to return from the lower part of your body to the central circulatory system. Otherwise, you could find yourself dizzy, light-headed or worse. Slow down your pace for about five minutes to allow your heart rate to decrease. More than one person has had tragic results by not allowing themselves this cool-down period after exercise. The case of Barbara illustrates this necessity dramatically. Barbara had just returned from an early morning jog. She jogged right into her bathroom to take a shower and turned the hot water on strong. Before she could adjust the temperature, she had passed out in the tub under the scalding water. Barbara ended up in the hospital with second degree burns over most of her body. (Some people have keeled over with cardiac arrest—Barbara was lucky.) In summary, we can't stress too strongly—warm up, do, but underdo (at least at first), and cool down.

HOW MUCH TIME DO I NEED TO SPEND EXERCISING?

This will depend on the intensity of your exercise and type of exercise you choose. You will spend more calories when you do high intensity exercises, such as running or cross country skiing, than you will when you do lower intensity exercises, like walking or biking. Exercising for 20-30 minutes, three or four days per week, is usually recommended for increasing cardiovascular fitness. For fat/weight loss, the long term goal is to exercise for five or six days per week for 50-60 minutes at a lower level of intensity (65-70 percent of maximum heart rate).

WHAT TYPE OF EXERCISE DO I CHOOSE?

Again, we recommend consulting your doctor. You may have some physical problems which need to be taken into account before you become the triathlete of the year. However, most physicians believe walking, exercise bicycling, and swimming can't be beat. Walking or cycling at a slow pace for a short period of time is safe for most people. If you have joint problems, swimming or water exercises (you don't need to know how to swim or even get your hair wet) are recommended. For fat loss, walking, bicycling and running have been found to be the most

16

effective.

We have given you a brief look at the FITT principle concepts. In the next few chapters we will help you set up your exercise program and get started with it.

IN A NUTSHELL
1. Monitor your pulse or employ the talking pace test.
2. Do, but underdo!
3. Warm up and cool down.

CHAPTER 5

LIFTING OFF!

One of the thorniest problems the beginning exerciser has is getting started. Many have wished for the magic exercise that requires no personal effort, but to date none has been found effective, at least for aerobic fitness and weight loss. So you're back to relying on your own efforts. No one else can work those muscles for you but you.

What is this thing called "fitness"? According to the President's Council on Physical Fitness, it is defined as the ability to carry out daily tasks with vigor and alertness, without undue fatigue and with ample energy to enjoy leisure time pursuits and to meet unforeseen emergencies. Furthermore, regardless of age, achieving physical fitness will improve the capacity of your heart and lungs for work, change your body composition, improve the flexibility, strength and endurance of your muscles and improve your emotional stability (not to mention your self esteem). Other benefits are that you will become more agile, have better balance and coordination, be quicker and stronger and react faster. Also recent studies indicate you will live a longer and better quality life.

THE CHOICE IS YOURS!

Now is the time for you to answer the question, "Am I willing to make a commitment to achieving this goal (becoming fit)?" If you answered "yes" to this question, read on. Making this commitment means you are ready to change certain aspects of your life to accommodate some new habits of exercise. New habits of any type are not acquired just by wishing. New habits are acquired by deciding how the habit will benefit you, what you are going to do, when you are going to do it, where you are going to do it, how you are going to do it, and, lastly, to actually do it.

WHAT ABOUT YOU?

Take a few minutes to answer the following questions about you and fitness.

1. What are your reasons for making a commitment to fitness at this time in your life?

Do the costs outweigh the benefits? The following analysis may help you decide.

FOR ME:

Benefits Of Not Exercising	Benefits Of Exercising
Costs Of Exercising	Costs Of Not Exercising

What did you decide?

2.   What type of exercise are you considering doing? Examine the pros and cons of each type.

3.   When are you planning to work exercise into your schedule? How long will you plan to exercise at first?

4.   Where are you going to do your exercise?

To help you give some preliminary thought to why, what, when and where, let's take the case of Sherry.

THE CASE OF SHERRY
Answering all of the above questions doesn't guarantee success. Sherry's situation is a case in point. Sherry considered herself a failure in her quest for fitness. She had made the choice and commitment; she

knew why and she thought she knew what, where and when. Sherry was in her early fifties and believed she was overweight. During the summer, she chose fitness as a means of preventing osteoporosis and for weight management, as well as overall well-being. Her plan included a twenty minute walk three times a week in her neighborhood after work. This plan went well until she had major surgery in the late fall. Her surgery was followed by the holiday season and a long vacation trip. When she was ready to resume her exercise in February, she had the same plan in mind. Unfortunately, this time she was unable to carry it out and didn't know why she was unable to motivate herself to begin again.

Many people would have quit when they thought they had failed, but Sherry was determined to form more positive health habits. In analyzing what had gone wrong with her plan, she found she was reluctant to walk by herself after dark. After she realized there was simply a glitch in her plan and not in herself, we were able to explore alternative courses of action that would stand a chance of success. Brainstorming for new options allowed Sherry to choose from several alternatives. Among these options were to use the stationary bicycle she had at home or exercise with television programs. She might have purchased video-taped exercise programs, a treadmill, a cross-country skiing device, or a rowing machine. If she wanted to get by cheaply, she could have walked in a shopping mall or used a mini-trampoline. Lastly, she could have joined a health club.

Sherry would have been no better off if she picked one of these alternatives without examining the pros and cons of each. Many fitness programs have bitten the dust because the exercise chosen was unrealistic. The first alternative she examined was whether or not to ride her stationary bicycle. Once before, she had determined that this would be her chosen mode of exercise, but had given up after a short time because the seat was too uncomfortable and the bicycle was in the basement facing a brick wall. Budding exercise enthusiasts will seldom continue a program if it is too uncomfortable or too boring. Had Sherry traded in her too small seat for a larger, more comfortable model and placed her bicycle in a room with a television set and/or reading stand, she might have enjoyed it more. At this time, Sherry had built up an aversion to the bicycle; therefore, she decided it would not be a realistic choice for her.

OTHER OPTIONS

Treadmills, cross-country skiing machines, rowing machines, and stair-climbing machines require a significant investment and can take up significant amounts of living space. Although Sherry did not rule out these alternatives altogether, they were not realistic for her at this time. She is contemplating renting one or more of these for a future trial. She rejected the mini-trampoline because she had heard an exercise physiologist discuss the risk of injuries associated with this equipment.

Health clubs require a greater expenditure of time and money than do home exercise programs. Few of us can afford the two to three hours per day commitment of time that is required for going to a health club, suiting up for exercise, exercising, showering, dressing and driving home. Sherry did not believe she had this much time to commit. Another consideration is that the dues at most health clubs are several hundred dollars per year—about the cost of a good piece of home exercise equipment.

On the other hand, if someone needs to get out of the house, like a mom home with small children all day, a health club can provide many positive benefits, such as socializing with other adults. Our point is that each person needs to weigh all the pros and cons based on his or her own situation.

Sherry decided after debating the above alternatives that she would purchase a low impact aerobic videotape. She did, and reported at our next meeting that she had gotten started and had met her objective of exercising three times each week. Her plan was to continue with the aerobic videotape.

However, at the following visit, Sherry was back to thinking she had failed again. She had loaned her VCR to her daughter for a couple of weeks and had not been able to carry out her chosen plan. The problem this time was lack of a backup plan. Sherry could have gone to the shopping center and walked, even though this activity would not have been her first choice. In fact, she had taken a short walk on her lunch hour with a coworker, but had discounted this as an exercise.

For an exercise program to succeed, you need to have not only Plan A, but also Plan B and perhaps Plan C. Plans B and C may not be your most favorite activities, but at least they will enable you to stay on your path to fitness when Plan A is temporarily disrupted.

GIVE YOURSELF A BREAK!

Don't think you are a failure if your plan doesn't work. All this means is that you need to go back to the drawing board and see why it didn't work and keep trying out different plans until you find one that fits you and your special needs. Sherry finally believes that she will be successful. And we agree because she now knows that she must take into account not only why and what she is going to do for exercise, but also when and where she can get the job done consistently.

Some words you always should remember never to say are "always", "never", and "should". More new habits are trashed by a part of us rebelling against you saying to yourself, "Well, I should exercise today. I said I would always exercise on Mondays and never skip a session." And, when you don't exercise every Monday, you feel guilty and say things to yourself, like "I'm a failure" or, "I've never succeeded, why should I succeed this time?" Before you know it, you have beaten up on yourself to the point that you say, "Well, I've blown it, what's the use?" A positive motto to remember here is **"PROGRESS, NOT PERFECTION."** No one we know behaves perfectly all the time. We have found our clients succeed when they make their exercise habit a choice. Once you have made a commitment to exercise, there are days when you will not feel like meeting your goal. When this happens, choose to postpone it for a day.

If you feel yourself slipping in your resolve for more than a few days, go back to your **FOR ME** analysis of the costs and benefits of exercising and see if your reasons are still worthwhile for you to continue the fitness choice. If the cost of continuing to exercise at this time in your life is too much, you can choose to stop. Perhaps you will feel like making the choice for fitness again at a later date. If your choice is to stop exercising, then it is pointless to feel guilty about it. Keep in mind that it may take six months or longer before you become "hooked" on the exercise habit and what works for friends and relatives may not work for you.

DO I NEED TO KEEP A DIARY OF MY EXERCISE?

We certainly recommend it! Most new habits require several weeks, if not months, of continual reinforcement to stand a chance of becoming permanent. One of the most reinforcing things you can do is to keep a record of your achievements, whether you are acquiring new exercise habits or new eating habits. If you are getting discouraged, you can look back at where you started and see how far you have come. As you begin to get more fit, your resting pulse will usually drop; this can be a very tangible measure of your progress. Take your resting pulse before you get out of bed in the morning.

GETTING STARTED

To help you get started, use the following exercise worksheet. (Make extra copies as necessary.

EXERCISE WORKSHEET: PLAN AND DIARY

WEEK NO.: _____ DATES OF WEEK: _____ WEEKLY GOAL: _____

Day	✓When Completed	Planned Time(s)	Activity	Exercise Heart Rate	Distance/ Duration	Comments
Monday						
Tuesday						
Wednesday						
Thursday						
Friday						
Saturday						
Sunday						

RESTING PULSE (Take Once A Week):

PLANNING: For best results in forming an exercise habit, jot down in pencil which days and times you are planning to exercise this week. Consult your calendar to see if what you are planning is realistic and then make any necessary changes in your plan. When you follow your plan, simply make a check mark beside the completed exercise time. If you need to deviate from your plan, write down what you actually did in ink. Treat your planned exercise time as you would an appointment. Remember to mark it on your regular scheduling calendar also.

EXCEPTIONS TO THE RULE!

The best laid plans often go astray, including exercise plans. Vacations, illness, change of season, change in jobs and/or schedules, change in your children's schedules, visiting family or friends, change in family situations (marriage, divorce, death, income, retirement) can have an impact on your exercise schedule. When possible, plan ahead, but don't let a temporary setback get in the way of your achieving your long range goal—to be fit. Alter your plans or make new plans as soon as possible. And, if you have to stop for awhile, simply plan to resume as soon as you can. You can maintain your current level of fitness with as few as two 10-15 minute exercise periods per week. You probably won't improve, but you won't lose much ground either.

IN A NUTSHELL
1. Examine all angles, plus the costs and benefits to you before making your commitment to exercise.
2. Keeping a diary helps.
3. Making a basic plan along with backup plans is essential.

Chapter 6

FUEL FOR FITNESS

Before we go into the food section of this book, let's talk about how to fuel this fit body of yours. The fuel we get from food is in the form of carbohydrate (starches and sugars), protein (meat, fish, poultry, milk, cheese, legumes), and fat (oil, margarine, butter, salad dressings, etc.) which are our primary sources of calories. Our bodies are burning calories twenty-four hours per day. How many, at any particular time, depends on what we are doing. The more active we are, the more calories we burn. Carbohydrate and fat calories are the main sources of fuel. Protein is necessary to build and maintain our muscle mass, but can also be used for fuel if not enough of the other sources are on hand. Any calories we don't use are stored in the body as fat. If your goal is to reduce these stores of body fat, the type and intensity of exercise is crucial, as well as the type of fuel you consume.

For those of you who are "going for the gold" (fat loss), an hour a day is the price we pay—five or six times per week of low intensity exercise (at the lower end of your target heart rate range).

WHY IS THIS PRICE SO HIGH?

It has to do with body fitness and the fuel your muscles burn during exercise. The more fit your body, the more efficiently your muscles will burn fat as a primary fuel. It takes a low intensity exercise period of about one hour to achieve maximum use of body fat to fuel the exercise. And, isn't this the point—less fat?

WHY DO I NEED CARBOHYDRATE?

Aerobic exercise needs glucose (blood sugar) as a starter fuel. Our bodies prepare for this by storing glucose in the liver and muscles in long chains called glycogen (a starch). When you eat carbohydrate in adequate amounts—now believed to be at least 55-60 percent of your total calories—your body will store glycogen. If you do not take in enough carbos from your food, the body is likely to get it from breaking down protein, either from your dietary protein intake or—heaven forbid—from your own body protein (muscles and organs), in order to obtain the glucose it needs for fuel. Glucose is essential for us to perform our daily activities. The brain does not function well at all without it. Some authorities compare the function of glucose in the burning of fat to the use of kindling in starting a fire. Your fire will burn better with a kindling primer, just as your fat stores will burn better if you have enough glucose to act as your "fat kindling".

WHAT IS ALL THIS ABOUT A MORE FIT BODY BEING ABLE TO STORE MORE GLUCOSE?

The more well trained your muscles are, the more glycogen (glucose) they can store. For this reason, people who train for marathons can go long periods of time on their body stores of fuel. The unfit, untrained body will "run out of gas" after a very short time because it will not have very adequate stores of glycogen. We urge you to start an exercise program because only exercise will give you well trained muscles.

WHY DO ALL THESE POPULAR REDUCING DIETS TELL ME TO EAT VERY LITTLE OR NO CARBOHYDRATE AND YOU ARE TELLING ME TO EAT A LOT?

Most veteran dieters believe carbohydrate foods are fattening. Nothing is farther from the truth. The reason these diet programs have you drop carbos from your menu is that the muscles in your body can store about a pound of glycogen. It takes almost three pounds of water to assist in this storage. Lower your glycogen stores by dropping carbos from your diet and you will experience an immediate drop in weight of several pounds. Then, when you begin to restock your muscle glycogen cupboards, you will regain this lost water weight. Your immediate thought is that starchy foods are fattening. They caused you to gain weight, didn't they?

Actually, per gram, carbohydrate has 4 calories; protein, 4 calories; fat, 9 calories; and alcohol, 7 calories. One teaspoon will hold about 5 grams, so you can see that one teaspoon of sugar has 20 calories while a teaspoon of oil has about 45 calories. We used to say a calorie is a calorie whatever its source, but recent studies indicate that calories from fat are more fattening than the calories from carbohydrate. It seems that as our bodies are processing our food, only 75 percent of unneeded calories from carbohydrate are converted to stored body fat, while 97 percent of unneeded fat calories are stored as body fat.

IN A NUTSHELL
1. Your body needs carbohydrate for maximum performance.
2. Because fat appears more fattening, decreasing fat in the diet holds the most promise for lowering body fat levels.

Chapter 7

FERRET OUT THOSE FATS!

Now that you know fat is potentially more fattening than carbohydrate and that the amount of fat in the diet is closely related to the amount of fat on the frame, are there other reasons to be concerned about the amount of fat you eat? Yes, whether you are lowering fat in your diet as a body fat or weight management tool, there are many other reasons to be interested in a reduced fat intake. Perhaps you are concerned about preventing certain health problems which have been associated with eating a high fat diet, or maybe your doctor has already prescribed a low fat diet to lower your cholesterol level. We will be discussing the use of lower fat food choices for cholesterol and for diabetes management after we finish our discussion of using a low fat diet as a body fat management tool.

If you are tired of calorie counting, lowering the amount of fat in the diet will almost automatically insure a lowered calorie intake, but without the pain of calorie counting.

Here's the scoop! We are going to show you an easy way to make informed healthy food choices by using fat grams.

WHERE DO I FIND THESE FAT GRAMS?

They can be found in the first column of the food tables, beginning on page 59. Remember, if you keep the total fat content low in your diet, you probably will have lowered the total number of calories you are eating. Since fat is the most concentrated form of calories and one of the least visible ones, knowing the fat content of the foods you eat can help you in substantially cutting calories without the hassle of counting them.

But you may be thinking, "Can I eat all the pure sugar foods such as some candies, sugars and soft drinks, or alcoholic beverages which do not have any fat content?"

We urge you to exercise common sense in the matter of the pure sugar foods and alcoholic beverages. If you do, it **is** possible to watch your fat intake only and eat a healthy diet while lowering calories without counting them. If you choose to eat unlimited amounts of these foods just because they do not contain fat, you could be kidding yourself. These foods contain few beneficial nutrients!

HOW MANY FAT GRAMS SHOULD I PLAN TO USE PER DAY?

A good rule of thumb is to aim for 35-50 or fewer fat grams per day if you are a woman and 40-60 if you are a man. You will most likely be consuming less fat than you are now as well as a healthier diet than you were before you started monitoring your fat intake.

If you want to be more precise and figure your fat grams based on

20-30% of your calorie needs, as most dietary guidelines suggest, then you will need to know what your estimated daily calorie needs are.

HOW DO I KNOW HOW MANY CALORIES I NEED?

You won't for sure, because your calorie needs are based primarily on the amount of your lean body mass. (See pages 2 and 3.) Even though you might know the weight of your lean body mass and your body fat percent, there are no easily used guidelines to help you figure your daily calorie needs using this information. Your calorie needs are also affected by your physical activity level and inherited factors.

We have chosen to base our calorie guidelines on information presented in the 1989 edition of *RECOMMENDED DIETARY ALLOWANCES*. These guidelines are based on people engaging in very light, sedentary activities. Your own calorie needs may vary. But for the purposes of figuring your desired fat intake, these guidelines are close enough. So here's a table to help you in computing daily calorie needs to arrive at your daily fat intake.

TABLE 7-1
CALORIES PER POUND BASED ON AGE

Ages 15-18	16
Ages 19-24	14
Ages 25-50	13
Ages 51+	12

For example, Connie, who is 40 and weighs 150 pounds, has an estimated calorie need of about 1950 calories per day. We arrived at this figure this way: 13 x 150 = 1950. Or, Max, who is 55 and weighs 175 pounds, needs 2100 calories (12 x 175 = 2100).

NOW THAT I HAVE ESTIMATED MY CALORIE NEEDS, HOW DO I FIGURE 20 OR 30% OF MY CALORIES AS FAT GRAMS?

It just so happens we have concocted an easy to use do-it-yourself table. See Table 7-2 on page 28.

TABLE 7-2
DAILY LEVELS OF CALORIES AND FAT
Fat Grams

Calories	(30%) Of Calories	(20%) Of Calories
1400	46	31
1500	50	33
1600	54	36
1700	56	38
1800	60	40
1900	64	42
2000	66	44
2100	70	47
2200	74	49
2300	78	51
2400	80	53
2500	84	56

For example, Connie sets 65 grams of fat as her daily intake if she is aiming for a fat intake of 30% of her estimated calorie needs. If she chooses to lower her fat intake to 20% of her calories, she will aim for about 43 grams of fat. Our advice is for you to begin at the 30% level and gradually reduce your fat intake to the 20% level if necessary.

WHAT ABOUT COUNTING CALORIES TO LOSE WEIGHT?

We don't advise it because we have found that lowering fat in the diet is usually enough for lowering fat in the body. Plus, if you don't count calories, you will avoid the physical and psychological effects of watching every bite you put in your mouth. However, we know there are a few calorie conscious diehards out there, so we have kept the calorie information in this edition of the book.

To lose weight, you will first need to estimate your calorie needs for keeping your weight where it is. Use Table 7-1 on page 27. View your estimated calorie needs as a ballpark figure. Remember, many people who are chronic dieters may have lowered their metabolic rates and may not need this many calories. Review Chapters One and Two of this book for more discussion of this problem.

There are about 3500 calories in one pound of fat. In theory then, to lose one pound of fat a week, subtract 500 calories a day from your estimated weight maintenance needs (3500 calories in one pound of fat divided by 7 days in a week). For example, you estimated your needs at 2000 calories per day to maintain your present weight. Your new calorie level would be 1500 calories to lose 1 pound in a week.

However, we advise using a more moderate approach, based on current knowledge. The people who have the most success keeping off their poundage maintain a permanent exercise habit, as we have discussed previously. For this reason, we advise gradually increasing your physical activity level by 30-60 minutes per day and lowering calories by only 250 per day. Remember, you can avoid the whole issue of counting calories by simply counting fat grams.

If you still insist on counting calories, there is an easier way. We use calorie points instead of calories because points are easier to count. Please read below to find out how to work with calorie points.

WHAT IS A CALORIE POINT?

A calorie point is approximately 75 calories. For instance, a 1500 calorie diet is 20 calorie points for the day. See the calorie point conversion table below for other calorie levels. We have also included fat gram levels that will amount to 20-30% of your daily calories.

After you have estimated your calorie points per day, you need to know how to choose foods that add up to that number. Look on page 59 for the **TABLE OF FOOD VALUES** where you will find calorie points listed for most foods.

WHY USE CALORIE POINTS?

Calorie points are less difficult to count than calories because it is easier to add 1 plus 1 instead of 63 and 86 calories. Counting calories can be very confusing, because not all the same foods appear to have been created equal so far as calorie counting books are concerned. For example, a large apple listed in one book might be 80 calories, in another 101 calories, and yet in a third, 123 calories. Also, adding figures such as 177 for 3 ounces of rump roast, 63 for a slice of bread, and 101 for an apple requires that most of us carry a calculator at all times. Isn't it easier to add 2.5 for the roast, 1 for the bread, and 1.5 for the apple?

TABLE 7-3
DAILY LEVELS OF CALORIE POINTS AND FAT GRAMS

Calories	Calorie Points	Fat Grams (30% of Calories)	(20% of Calories)
1400	18.5	46	31
1500	20	50	33
1600	21.5	54	36
1700	22.5	56	38
1800	24	60	40
1900	25.5	64	42
2000	26.5	66	44
2100	28	70	47
2200	29.5	74	49
2300	31	78	51
2400	32	80	53
2500	33.5	84	56

YOU DID NOT LIST THE LEVEL OF CALORIES I NEED EACH DAY. HOW CAN I FIGURE MY FAT GRAMS?

Let's assume your day's calorie needs are 2700. To figure the fat gram level for 30% of calories, multiply 2700 times .3—this equals 810 calories from fat. Then, divide 810 by 9 (there are 9 calories in each gram of fat). Your fat grams for the 30% level are 90. For 20% of your calories as fat, multiply 2700 times .2—this equals 540 calories from fat. Divide by 9 to find your fat gram total equals 60. For others of you whose calorie levels were not listed on our chart, you can plug your own numbers into the calculations above.

HOW CAN I LOWER FAT IN MY DIET WITHOUT COUNTING FAT GRAMS?

Some of you will do just as well making gradual changes in your diet and will be able to lower fat significantly by trying some of the "tricks" listed below without actually counting each and every fat gram that goes into your mouth. You might start out by writing down the foods you currently eat for a few days and look up the grams of fat you are presently consuming. Then, look at some of the ideas below for trimming the fat from your food and see what changes you are willing to make.

Bonnie, for instance, feels that looking up the foods she eats and counting fat grams is too much like all of the other times she has dieted. She did agree to write down her intake for a few days, and it became apparent that just by changing from a pint of regular premium ice cream to a pint of nonfat frozen yogurt per day that she could save a significant amount of fat and therefore, calories. She liked the frozen yogurt just as well as the ice cream so she did not feel she was making a sacrifice.

Bonnie may find other changes she can make without feeling she is giving up all that is near and dear to her heart.

EASY TRICKS TO LOWER FAT

INSTEAD OF THIS	TRY THIS
Whole milk or 2% fat milk	1% fat milk or skim milk
4% fat cottage cheese	1-2% fat cottage cheese
Regular cheeses	Reduced fat or no fat cheeses
Regular butter or margarine	Whipped or reduced fat margarine
Whipping cream	Reduced fat dessert topping or whipped evaporated skim milk
Cream in recipes	Evaporated skim milk
Sour cream	Non-fat plain yogurt
Fats and oils used for frying	Non-stick pan sprays
Cream sauces and gravies	Thicken skim milk or fat-free broth with cornstarch or other thickeners
Ice cream	Fat free frozen yogurt or fat free iced milk

INSTEAD OF THIS	TRY THIS
Butter, margarine, salad dressings and other fat seasonings for vegetables	Spice blends, seasoned pepper, herbs, spices, lemon juice, vinegar, fat-free broth, fat-free cheese, reduced fat or non-fat salad dressings
Potato chips, corn chips	Pretzels, low or non fat popcorn, fat-free corn chips
Regular ground beef	7-10% or less fat ground beef
Regular wieners	1 gram fat wieners
Regular luncheon meats	3% or less fat luncheon meats
Beef, pork, lamb and veal	Lean, well trimmed cuts 3-4 times per week, fish, skinless poultry and legumes more often

Check the food tables in the last half of this book for more options.

WHAT HAPPENS IF I OVERDO? WILL I RUIN MY CHANCES FOR SUCCESS?

We suggest viewing your intake by the week instead of the day. Some days you may be under your level of fat grams and/or calorie points. Because of this, if you run over a few grams every now and then, don't worry. Some people add up their grams of fat for the week and divide by 7. If this average figure is within a gram or two of your daily goal, consider your goal to be met. If you are consistently over, analyze what is contributing to this and make plans to alter some aspect of your intake. For example, if you find that you are spending 38 of your 50 fat grams on a McD.L.T. and French Fries, ask yourself what alternative McDonald's has that you like as well and that has fewer fat points. Or, look at the choices of the other restaurants for lower fat alternatives. Some of you may choose to brown bag your lunch to save fat grams to spend more on favorite foods for breakfast or dinner. When you use the information in the food tables to make informed choices, you can nearly always find something you like just as well or almost as well as some of the higher fat choices. Our motto has always been **"THERE ARE NO INAPPROPRIATE FOODS—THERE MAY BE INAPPROPRIATE AMOUNTS!"** Recall our other motto from the chapters on exercise because it applies here too—**"PROGRESS, NOT PERFECTION!"**

REMEMBER, USE THE TABLE OF FOOD VALUES FOR MAKING INFORMED CHOICES OF FOODS.

We have not included all this information to make your life harder. Rather, you are now in a position of being able to make your own food choices because you have the information yourself. This way, you do not need to depend on a diet sheet or your dietitian or doctor to tell you what you can and can't do. With fat grams, just as with calorie points, you probably will do a bit of averaging. That is, some days you will be under your goal and some days you will be over it. As long as you have decreased your fat intake overall, you should improve your chances of preventing heart disease and/or cancer. If you have diabetes, it will be better controlled. Enjoy!

RECORD AS YOU GO!

If you're like most of us, you'll develop a severe case of amnesia two hours after a meal. Keeping records at the time of eating, even if it's only a simple tally of your fat grams, is a big help. The food diary helps in several ways. It can be a big awareness booster about what you are eating. More important though, a record of any new habit acts as a reinforcer in the establishment of the habit, whether it is an exercise or an eating habit or any other habit you are trying to cultivate. Also, we have found that the diary can help absolve some of the guilt feelings people have about consuming certain types of foods. When you have a diary, you can look back at it and see that you have not in fact overeaten, even though you felt you had. We suggest making copies of the sample food diary which follows.

FOOD DIARY

Time	Food	Amount	Fat Grams	Calorie Points	Sodium Points	Fiber Grams Total/Soluble

Physical Activity   **Other Habits**

SOMETIMES MY WEIGHT GOES UP FOR NO GOOD REASON AND IT CAUSES ME TO THINK "WHAT'S THE USE, NOTHING WORKS!"

Many times people give up when they are doing everything right and still do not get the reward (weight loss, or at least not a weight gain) they feel they deserve for all the effort they have put into their habit changes. Sometimes it pays to play detective. Inspect your medicine closet. Some medicines you take may cause you to have extra fluid weight. Ask your dietitian or doctor about any medicines you are taking. In fact, some medicines cause an increase in appetite and eating with a resultant weight gain. It pays to know the effect any medicines you are taking have on weight.

Even a meal with a high salt content can result in a temporary fluid increase of three or four or more pounds. And, speaking of water weight—women, don't push the panic button if you gain a few pounds of fluid close to your menstrual period or at the time you ovulate. Some people gain as many as eight or more pounds at the time of their period which drop quickly once the period is finished. It is not uncommon for even the most slim person to feel fat at the time of her menstrual period. It is not uncommon either for most women to have an increased appetite before their menstrual periods begin. It may help your morale to keep a graph of your own weight changes so that you can predict when these increases in weight will occur.

IN A NUTSHELL

1. Find out how many fat grams are healthy for you to eat in a day.
2. Count fat grams instead of calories to lower your body fat.
3. Use the EASY TRICKS TO LOWER FAT if you want **really** easy ways to lower fat in your diet.
4. Keep a log of your fat intake.

Chapter 8

HOW TO SUCCEED WHILE REALLY TRYING!

We thought it might be helpful to recap some tips about maintaining your new healthy habits—exercising and eating more fiber and carbohydrates and less fat. We have dropped some hints along the way and felt that collecting them together along with a few new ones would help you in your quest for success.

1. MODESTY BECOMES YOU!
Setting realistic, achievable goals is the first hallmark of success. The second is being able to evaluate your goals and set new ones if the old ones don't work. Turn mistakes into a learning experience rather than bashing yourself with the old failure "tapes".

2. FIND OUT HOW FAT YOU ARE.
Knowing how fat you are is the first step in helping you set realistic eating and exercise goals.

3. LISTEN TO AND GET TO KNOW YOUR BODY.
Eat when you are physically hungry and not for some of the other reasons people eat such as boredom, anger, depression, habit, time of day, etc. To eat when you are physically hungry, you need to recognize symptoms of physical hunger. These might be a growling stomach, headache, shakiness, tiredness, and sometimes anxiety (not situational).

When it comes to exercise, do, but don't overdo. Know when to take a day off or when to stop your exercise session. If you feel very tired and don't know if you should go ahead and exercise, start slowly for 10 minutes. If you do not feel better after 10 minutes, give yourself permission to stop. If you do feel better, carry on!

4. EAT AT LEAST THREE WELL-BALANCED MEALS A DAY.
Eating regularly and not skipping meals is a good way to avoid food cravings and possibly bingeing. High carbohydrate and fiber containing foods such as starchy foods, fruits and vegetables are particularly helpful.

Some researchers have found that a carbohydrate snack in late afternoon serves most of us well and can help us avoid overeating at dinner and at night. Many of our clients who have followed this advice were able to stop overeating at night.

5. PLEASE DON'T VIEW YOUR NEW EXERCISE AND EATING GOALS AS JUST ANOTHER REDUCING DIET OR PROGRAM.
Dieting means deprivation, physical and psychological, and almost always assures you will end up fatter and feeling like a failure.

6. KEEP A LOG OF BOTH YOUR EXERCISE AND EATING HABITS.

Keeping a log is a good reinforcer of new habits and can help you in evaluating when or if you need to set different goals.

7. PROGRESS, NOT PERFECTION.

View any lapses, not as failures, but as learning experiences. Focus on what you have done, rather than what you have not done.

8. POSTPONE; DON'T SAY "NO, I CAN'T HAVE IT" .

If you forbid yourself to eat a desired food, you will end up obsessing about it and ultimately eat more than would have satisfied you originally. There's a part of us that doesn't want to be told "No".

Instead of saying "No", which almost guarantees you'll eat it anyway, try saying, "I'll wait until after this TV show finishes, and if I still want it, I will have some." Often, you will have forgotten about it by the time the show is over.

9. IF YOUR FRIENDS ARE JEALOUS OF YOUR SUCCESS AND TRY TO SABOTAGE YOU, YOU MAY WISH TO WIDEN YOUR CIRCLE OF ACQUAINTANCES.

Whether or not a person is successful in adopting permanent new habits can be predicted by whether or not they have supportive family and friends. If you are unable to change your family/friends, then learn to be assertive about your own needs. Also learning to tune out harmful (and often well-meant) remarks helps.

10. WHETHER OR NOT YOU CHANGE YOUR FOOD HABITS, EXERCISE, EXERCISE, EXERCISE!

Research shows that people who maintain consistent exercise habits are those most likely to maintain lower body fat levels.

Chapter 9

FIRST YOU SAY WE CAN AND THEN WE CAN'T
(Or, How to Sort Out the Conflicting Information Regarding Controlling Blood Cholesterol)

I NEED TO WATCH MY CHOLESTEROL AND SATURATED FAT INTAKE, BUT DON'T REALLY KNOW WHAT THESE TERMS MEAN.

No problem. Just remember that cholesterol is a waxy, fat-like substance found **only** in animal foods. It is essential for many body functions. And, even if you didn't eat any cholesterol, your liver would make enough for your body's needs. Saturated fat, on the other hand, is found in foods of both animal and plant origins. Generally, saturated fat is not liquid at room temperature.

WHY DO I NEED TO BE CONCERNED ABOUT CHOLESTEROL AND SATURATED FAT INTAKE?

A high blood level of cholesterol is a major contributor to developing hardening of the arteries (collections of hardened fat, cholesterol and debris in the inner walls of the arteries.) This condition, called atherosclerosis, can lead to heart attacks or strokes. High levels of cholesterol and saturated fat in the diet do tend to increase blood levels of cholesterol in some people. However, a high saturated fat intake is the biggest culprit in causing cholesterol levels to increase.

I AM SO CONFUSED ABOUT WHAT I CAN AND CAN'T EAT TO HELP LOWER THE CHOLESTEROL IN MY BLOOD.

We don't blame you. Many health professionals feel exactly the same way. The flood of current research, instead of clearing up our confusion, only seems to add to it. Several years back we were recommending that people increase the amount of polyunsaturated fatty acids (PUFAs) in their diet to lower their blood cholesterol. These PUFAs are found in oils such as safflower, sunflower, and corn. And people went around dutifully adding several teaspoons per day of these oils to their food.

The monounsaturated fatty acids (MUFAs) were thought to have no effect on cholesterol levels in the blood. MUFAs are found in canola, olive and peanut oils. One more group of fatty acids that had a "bad" reputation were the saturated fatty acids (SFAs) found in animal foods and tropical oils such as palm, palm kernel and coconut. SFAs and dietary cholesterol itself were blamed for increasing the level of cholesterol in the blood. So diets were restricted in cholesterol and the SFAs. Since the so-called red meats and dairy products contained high levels of SFAs and cholesterol, they were severely limited or banned. Tropical oils (coconut, palm, etc.) were also prohibited, and shellfish were a "NO-NO" because of an apparent high cholesterol content.

More recently, we have been recommending the use of oils high in MUFAs for cooking because some research indicated MUFAs helped lower total cholesterol in the blood without lowering the "good" cholesterol known as high density lipoproteins (HDLs). PUFAs lowered total cholesterol but appeared to lower the "good" HDLs.

Now we are hearing that neither the PUFAs nor MUFAs lower the "good" HDLs. Furthermore, the tropical oils and some SFAs may not be the bad guys they are made out to be. Some authorities contend that dietary cholesterol may or may not affect blood cholesterol, depending on the individual's response to it.

Shellfish are back on the menu because chemical analyses have become more precise and the cholesterol content was not as high as was first thought.

IN THE MIDST OF ALL THIS CONFUSION, WHAT DO I DO?

We support the dietary guidelines from such prestigious health organizations as the American Heart Association, the American Cancer Society, the American Diabetes Association, and the American Dietetic Association to lower total fat in the diet to 20-30% of calories. The reason these and other health organizations believe we need to be more stingy with fat in our diets is that certain forms of heart disease and cancers have been associated with a high fat intake. We also know that most people with diabetes can better control their diabetes if they decrease dietary fat.

This reduction in fat will automatically reduce your intake of all fatty acids. We also feel confident that until the research dust settles, limiting intake of foods high in SFAs is a good idea. See table 9-4 on page 42 for fatty acid content of foods. As far as the level of cholesterol in the diet is concerned, we will stay with the American Heart Association's recommendation of 300 or fewer milligrams of dietary cholesterol per day.

We believe you can achieve your health goals by lowering your intake of fat (with or without tedious calorie counting), minimizing sugar and alcohol intake and eating a diet high in fiber and complex carbohydrates.

WHAT IS A GOOD LEVEL FOR MY CHOLESTEROL?

Excellent question—everyone should know what their cholesterol reading is, including young people. The following table will help you know how you stand.

TOTAL CHOLESTEROL LEVELS		
DESIRABLE	**BORDERLINE–HIGH**	**TOO HIGH**
Less than 200 mg /dl	200-239 mg/dl	Over 239 mg/dl

Even more important than total cholesterol level is the ratio of your

HDLs to that total. For example, Max had a total cholesterol of 250 mg/dl, but his HDL level was 80 mg/dl for a ratio of 3.1. (divide the total cholesterol by the amount of the HDL). A desirable ratio is 4.5 or below. The best ratios are 3.5 or below. His doctors patted him on the back and told him he was in good shape. The point is, it is **not** enough to know only the total cholesterol figure. You need to find out your HDL and your low density lipoprotein (LDL) levels too.

The **higher** your level of HDL cholesterol, (the right stuff), the **lower** your risk of heart disease. The **higher** your LDL level, (the wrong stuff), the **greater** your risk of heart disease.

LDL CHOLESTEROL LEVELS		
DESIRABLE	**BORDERLINE–HIGH**	**TOO HIGH**
Less than 130 mg/dl	130-159 mg/dl	160 mg /dl or more

LDL levels are lowered by decreasing cholesterol and saturated fat intake in the diet. HDL levels are increased by exercising, quitting smoking, and losing weight.

When you eat a diet low in total fat, your cholesterol and saturated fat intake are decreased automatically. It is usually enough just to count total fat grams in your diet and follow the guidelines presented throughout this chapter.

BUT I WOULD LIKE TO KNOW WHAT IT ACTUALLY MEANS TO HAVE A 20 TO 30% FAT INTAKE.

We know some of you who started at the beginning of the book already know what is meant by a 20-30% intake of fat. However, for those of you who are just interested in lowering your blood cholesterol and may have started the book with this chapter, we will repeat this information here.

Because most people do not go around with a dietitian in their hip pocket, this guideline to lower fat to 20 or 30 percent of calories can be a confusing one; most dietitians would prefer not to be bothered with all of these mathematical computations either.

Look no further! Help is at hand! You do not need to be a math whiz to be able to eat the recommended level of fat in your diet.

A good rule of thumb is to aim for 35-50 or fewer fat grams per day if you are a woman and 40-60 if you are a man. You will most likely be consuming a lower fat and healthier diet than you are now.

If you want to be more precise and figure your fat grams based on 20-30% of your calorie needs, as most dietary guidelines suggest, then you will need to know what your estimated daily calorie needs are.

HOW DO I KNOW HOW MANY CALORIES I NEED?

You won't know for sure because your calorie needs are influenced by your physical activity level and inherited factors.

We have chosen to base our calorie guidelines on information presented in the 1989 edition of *RECOMMENDED DIETARY ALLOWANCES*. These guidelines are based on people engaging in very light, sedentary activities. Your own calorie needs may vary. But for the purposes of figuring your desired fat intake, these guidelines are close enough. So here's a table to help you in computing daily calorie needs to arrive at your daily fat intake.

TABLE 9-1
CALORIES PER POUND BASED ON AGE

Ages 15-18	16
Ages 19-24	14
Ages 25-50	13
Ages 51+	12

For example, Connie, who is 40 and weighs 150 pounds, has an estimated calorie need of about 1950 calories per day. We arrived at this figure this way: 13 x 150 = 1950. Or, Max, who is 55 and weighs 175 pounds, needs 2100 calories (12 x 175 = 2100).

You will need to find the number of calories per pound opposite your age and multiply this number times your weight in pounds.

DOES THIS MEAN I HAVE TO COUNT CALORIES, TOO?

No! You only did this calculation so you could figure your desirable number of fat grams per day. It just so happens we have concocted an easy to use "do-it-yourself" table. See below.

TABLE 9-2
DAILY LEVELS OF CALORIES AND FAT

Calories	Fat Grams	
	(30% of Calories)	(20% of Calories)
1400	46	31
1500	50	33
1600	54	36
1700	56	38
1800	60	40
1900	64	42
2000	66	44
2100	70	47
2200	74	49
2300	78	51

For example, Connie sets 65 grams of fat as her daily intake if she is aiming for a fat intake of 30% of her estimated calorie needs. If she chooses to lower her fat intake to 20% of her calories, she will aim for about 43 grams of fat. Our advice for you is to begin at the 30% level and gradually reduce your fat intake to the 20% level if necessary.

YOU DID NOT LIST THE LEVEL OF CALORIES I NEED EACH DAY. HOW CAN I FIGURE MY FAT GRAMS?

Let's assume your day's calorie needs are 2700. To figure the fat gram level for 30% of calories, multiply 2700 times .3—this equals 810 calories from fat. Then, divide 810 by 9 (there are 9 calories in each gram of fat). Your fat grams for the 30% level are 90. For 20% of your calories as fat, multiply 2700 times .2—this equals 540 calories from fat. Divide by 9 to find your fat gram total equals 60. For others of you whose calorie levels were not listed on our chart, you can plug your own numbers into the calculations above.

GUIDELINES TO LOWERING CHOLESTEROL IN THE DIET

When you look at the food tables, be aware that any food which is animal in origin, alone or in combination with other foods, has some cholesterol content. The potato, which has been seasoned with cheese or butter, is a good example. If the food is low in total fat content, it is probably no problem for you even if it contains some cholesterol. Exceptions include egg yolks and organ meats which are moderate in fat content but contain much more cholesterol than even red meat.

The American Heart Association has recommended keeping cholesterol intake below 300 milligrams per day. To accomplish this goal, use skim milk (even 1-2 percent milk has fat and cholesterol) and other low or no fat dairy products. Limit egg yolk intake to four per week and organ meat intake to one or fewer times per month. Keep intake of **lean** meat, fish or skinless poultry to four to six ounces per day.

To see if your cholesterol intake falls within these guidelines, use the chart below.

TABLE 9-3
CHOLESTEROL COMPARISON CHECK

FOOD	MILLIGRAMS OF CHOLESTEROL
Fruits, vegetables, grains	0
Nuts, seeds	0
Vegetable oils**	0
Egg whites	0
Skim milk or skim milk yogurt (1 cup)	4
Buttermilk (1 cup)	9
Whole milk (1 cup)	35
1 % fat cottage cheese (1 cup)	10
Creamed cottage cheese (1 cup)	31
Oysters, cooked (about 3.5 oz.)	45
Fish, lean or clams, cooked (about 3.5 oz.)	65
Chicken/turkey, light meat, cooked, without skin (about 3.5 oz.)	80

CHOLESTEROL COMPARISON CHECK

FOOD	MILLIGRAMS OF CHOLESTEROL
Chicken/turkey, dark meat, cooked, without skin (about 3.5 oz.)	95
Beef, lean, cooked (about 3.5 oz.)	**84**
Lobster, cooked (about 3.5 oz.)	85
Crab, cooked (about 3.5 oz.)	**100**
Pork, lean, cooked (about 3.5 oz.)	111
Mozzarella, part skim (1 oz.)	**17**
Shrimp, cooked (about 3.5 oz.)	150
Cheddar cheese (1 oz.)	**30**
Cream cheese (1 oz.)	31
Egg yolk (1 yolk)	**211**
Heavy whipping cream (1/4 cup)	82
Beef liver, cooked (about 3.5 oz.)	**389**
Chicken livers, cooked (about 3.5 oz.)	631
Beef kidney, cooked (about 3.5 oz.)	**700**
Butter (1 oz.)	62

GUIDELINES TO LOWER SATURATED FAT IN THE DIET

In general, choose polyunsaturated or monounsaturated oils or fats which are liquid at room temperature. On the label, look for the word *hydrogenated*, which means that a polyunsaturated vegetable fat has been turned into a partially saturated fat by adding hydrogen. In addition, until further research is in, beware of three liquid vegetable fats: coconut, palm and palm kernel oil. These are naturally highly saturated fats and are frequently used in the preparation of many convenience and fast foods. Cereals, crackers, microwave popcorn, and many frozen ready-to-heat products are some of the most notorious sources of these oils. **READ LABELS!!!**

When you do decide to use fat, some choices are better than others. Mono and polyunsaturated fats such as olive, canola, safflower or sunflower oil, along with corn oil, are the best choices. Other good oils are cottonseed, sesame seed, and soybean. Use a light hand when adding any fat to your cooking. You may find you have exceeded your fat gram goal. See the chart on the next page for comparing types of fats.

TABLE 9-4
OILS AND FATS—KNOW THE DIFFERENCES!!!

The fatty acid values are given as percentages of total fat and may not add up to 100 percent due to the presence of other fat substances in the oil.

Type of Fat or Oil	Percent of Fatty Acids In		
	Polyunsaturated	Monounsaturated	Saturated
Safflower Oil	74%	12%	9%
Sunflower Oil	65%	20%	10%
Corn Oil	59%	24%	13%
Soybean Oil	58%	24%	14%
Cottonseed Oil	52%	18%	26%
Canola Oil	30%	59%	7%
Olive Oil	8%	73%	13%
Peanut Oil	32%	46%	17%
Soft Tub Margarine, Typical	61%	18%	16%
Stick Margarine, Typical	32%	45%	18%
Vegetable Shortening	14%	51%	30%
Palm Oil	10%	37%	49%
Coconut Oil	2%	6%	87%
Palm Kernel Oil	2%	11%	82%
Cocoa Butter	3%	33%	60%
Tuna Fat	63%	?-	27%
Turkey Fat	23%	43%	30%
Chicken Fat	21%	45%	30%
Goose Fat	11%	57%	27%
Duck Fat	13%	49%	34%
Lard	11%	45%	39%
Mutton Fat	8%	41%	48%
Beef Fat	4%	41%	50%
Butter Fat	5%	30%	62%

Notice that the fats with the highest percentages of saturated fatty acids, the "bad" stuff, are listed toward the bottom of the chart. The worst animal fat offenders appear to be mutton, beef, and butter fat (found in full fat dairy products). Don't get dairy products with butter fat confused with low fat or fat free dairy products such as skim milk and fat free cheese and yogurt. These foods are necessary for a good diet.

To complicate the controversies surrounding MUFAs, PUFAs, and SFAs, there are also fatty acids known as "cis" and "trans". Margarines contain "trans" fatty acids due to the partial hydrogenation (saturation) process they undergo to keep them from being liquid oil. "Trans" fatty acids elevate blood LDL cholesterol. So what is a person to do, go back to butter? Until more facts are in, most experts believe margarine is still a better choice than butter. But, the moral to this story is, continue to follow a diet low in all types of fat.

I KEEP HEARING THAT OMEGA-3 OR EPA CAPSULES ARE A GOOD THING TO TAKE TO LOWER MY CHOLESTEROL.

Research shows that Eskimos who have a high intake of Omega-3 fatty acids (found in fish oils) have low cholesterol levels and a low incidence of heart disease. The effectiveness of EPA capsules in lowering cholesterol is not proven, and some authorities have found problems with their use. You certainly need to contact your physician before taking these capsules. Most experts believe that the best way for you to increase your intake of these important fatty acids is to eat two or more fish meals per week.

AND NOW FOR THE GOOD NEWS. . .

Another dietary goal aimed at helping you lower cholesterol in your blood is to eat more fiber and complex carbohydrates. Soluble fiber found in some cereals, fruits and vegetables, and mature **legumes** (such as dried beans, peas and lentils) is effective for most people in lowering cholesterol levels in the blood. For people with diabetes, foods high in soluble fiber have been found to be beneficial. Insoluble fiber is believed to be essential for good bowel health. Many authorities believe it may help prevent cancer of the bowel, as well as other problems such as hemorrhoids and diverticulosis. Remember, foods which are good sources of soluble and insoluble fiber are fruits, vegetables, legumes, and whole grain cereal products (most of these food groups are sources of complex carbohydrates). They are award winners since they contain few calories, lots of good nutrition, NO cholesterol, and practically no fat.

Based on his studies, fiber authority James W. Anderson, M.D., recommends 20-30 grams daily **total** plant fiber per intake of each 1000 calories. You need to include about 15-20 grams of soluble fiber each day. Dr. Anderson has given us permission to adapt his fiber tables from his book, **PLANT FIBER IN FOODS.** Check out your own intake using this table in Appendix B beginning on page 126. To have the desired positive effect on cholesterol or blood glucose (sugar), you will probably find yourself eating a lot of certain cereals and beans.

The following general guidelines may help you obtain the recommended plant fiber for the day:
● Starchy foods, preferably whole grain cereal products and breads (approximately 6-12 servings daily, depending on the number of calories consumed).
● Vegetables and fruits (5-13 servings daily—includes 1 serving of beans). OOPS, sorry, but fruit juices usually don't count as fiber sources.
● Inexperienced fiber eaters may want to ease into consuming all of the above recommended foods. Proceed cautiously! Fiber is famous for flatulence (intestinal gas)! You will feel better if you add one or two new foods at a time, rather than too much, too soon.

WARNING! You need plenty of water to prevent constipation on a high fiber diet—at least 6 to 8 glasses of liquids daily. Don't count on vegetable juices for much fiber. Some of the popular juicers remove much of the fiber during the juicing process.

It is very hard to mount up a significant tally of either calories or fat if you consume more fruits and foods high in complex carbohydrates (vegetables and starchy foods), especially if they are prepared without additional fat or sugar. For example, one puny 2 ounce candy bar contains 10 fat grams and 270 calories. For the same number of calories and **no** fat grams, you can have 1 apple, 1/2 cantaloupe, and 1 whole grapefruit. The candy bar is an example of a calorie dense food with few other redeeming features about it. With the fruit, you not only will feel stuffed, but you will have consumed generous amounts of fiber, vitamins, and minerals. As a matter of fact, some of the calories will never be absorbed because of the fiber content. We do not suggest that the fruit choice will always win out, but we urge you to give it a try, instead of the candy, at least some of the time.

Remember, it is one of the greatest myths of all time that starchy foods are fattening. Six regular sized slices of bread contain only about 400 calories. Six teaspoons of butter or margarine will add about 24 grams of fat and 215 calories. To save fat grams, one of the things we have done is to find a good tasting bread which is palatable without butter or margarine added to it and have learned to eat this bread plain. Even if you add a reduced sugar marmalade or jelly instead of the fat spread, you have saved more than 100 calories and used no fat grams.

WHAT IF MY TRIGLYCERIDES ARE HIGH TOO?

Triglycerides come from the fats in our foods and if blood levels are too high (above 200 mg/dl), you may be at risk for developing heart disease. Losing weight, lowering dietary fat, and eating more foods high in fiber and complex carbohydrates are the best things you can do to lower triglyceride levels—in other words, following the same guidelines that are recommended for lowering cholesterol.

Reducing intake of high sugar foods and alcoholic beverages usually helps also. Discuss your individual health concerns with your dietitian or physician.

LIFE AFTER FAT COOKING TIPS

Invest in the non stick varieties of skillets. Yes, they really do fry chicken without fat or flour. Use skillet or pan sprays to help avoid food sticking in any pan or skillet.

If you must use oil or fat, you'd be surprised how little you need. If a recipe calls for 2 tablespoons of fat, 1 teaspoon is enough to sauté your onions, garlic or whatever. Use vermouth or other dry white wine, burgundy, broth, tomato or vegetable juice cocktail for "sautéing" vegetables or meats. Add herbs and spices to your heart's content. "French fried" oven fried potato sticks are easier to prepare than regular deep fat fried ones. One teaspoon of oil sprinkled over 2 sliced potatoes on a cookie sheet will produce tasty "fries". Sprinkle with paprika and onion powder.

Try out this recipe. "Sauté" any vegetable or mix of vegetables such as zucchini squash, cherry tomatoes, onions, mushrooms, green peppers, broccoli, or carrot strips in 1/2 cup vermouth or burgundy, 1/4 teaspoon

44

of garlic powder and onion powder, and 1/2 teaspoon bouillon granules until the liquid is cooked down. Salt (if not restricted) and pepper to taste. Variation: Add soy sauce, lemon juice or Worcestershire Sauce in place of the bouillon.

PREPARING MEAT, POULTRY, FISH

Buy leaner cuts of meat such as rump roast or round steak. Trim off all visible fat from any cut before cooking. Skin all poultry BEFORE cooking. Buy water-packed tuna instead of oil packed. You'll save fat grams.

Pan-broil without fat. Use wine for cooking, if desired, unless you have a problem with alcohol. Cooking does evaporate some, but not all the alcohol, depending on the method of cooking.

Broiling in the oven or outdoors helps get rid of more fat. Marinades for barbecuing, broiling, or baking, which use lemon juice, wine, whiskey, vinegar, spices, and herbs tenderize and add flavor. Omit the oil or fat called for—you'll never miss it.

SAUCES, GRAVIES

Gravy can be made with any defatted meat broth and 2 table-spoons flour or corn starch dissolved in cold water and mixed with the simmering broth to make 1 cup. Before making a gravy, always let meat broth sit in the refrigerator until the fat comes to the top. Skim off. Use the same technique for sauces.

Can't throw out those leftovers? Try the best soup ever. This is one way to get rid of a habit many people have—cleaning up all the leftovers after a meal by eating them up themselves. So if you can't bring yourself to "waste" them instead of "waisting" them, try this. For those dibs and dabs of this and that which have been so tempting to eat instead of throwing out, start a soup pot in your freezer. Add that spoon of green beans, potatoes, any other vegetable, leftover meat broth, defatted meat scraps, rice, etc. which you can't bring yourself to part with. When you have enough scraps in your freezer container(s) for a meal, thaw, add broth or tomato juice, if necessary, and you will have some of the tastiest soup ever.

IN A NUTSHELL
1. Aim for a total blood cholesterol below 200 mg/dl.
2. A desirable ratio of HDL to total cholesterol is 4.5 or below.
3. Aim for a fat intake of no more than 20-30% of your calorie needs.
4. Consume more fats that are high in MUFAs and PUFAs such as olive, canola, sunflower, and corn oils.
5. Consume fewer foods high in saturated fats such as the tropical oils and most animal fats.
6. Eat more high fiber foods such as legumes, fruits, and vegetables.

Chapter 10

FOUNDATION FOR FITNESS

HOW CAN I BE SURE I AM EATING A NUTRITIOUS DIET?
Consult the **NUTRIENT INSURANCE GUIDE** below. Although it is not foolproof, you will be assured of meeting most of your nutrient requirements. We recommend eating at least the minimum number of servings of fruits and vegetables and whole grain breads and cereals, especially if you are to achieve a high fiber diet. Our **NUTRIENT INSURANCE GUIDE** is based on the new USDA's *The Food Guide Pyramid: A Guide to Daily Food Choices.*

NUTRIENT INSURANCE GUIDE
USE EACH DAY

6–11 servings of whole grain or enriched bread, cereal, cereal grains, pasta

3–5 servings of vegetables (Include at least 1 dark green or deep yellow vegetable)

2–4 servings of fruits (Include 1 citrus fruit or a good source of Vitamin C)

2 (2-3 ounce) servings of fish, poultry, meat, dried beans, eggs, nuts

2–3 servings of non-fat milk, yogurt, or low fat cheese

Some of you will find the following chart helpful in determining how many servings of each group to eat for different calorie levels.

NUMBER OF SERVINGS FOR VARIOUS CALORIE LEVELS

Food Group	Many Women Older Adults About 1600 Calories	Teenage Girls Active Women Most Men About 2200 Calories	Teenage Boys Active Men About 2800 Calories
Bread	6	9	11
Vegetable	3	4	5
Fruit	2	3	4
Milk**	2-3	2-3	2-3
Meat	2 (2.5 oz.)	2 (3 oz.)	2 (3.5 oz.)

If you choose low fat, lean foods from the major food groups and use fat, oils and sweets sparingly, you can eat the number of servings from each food group shown above.

**Women who are pregnant or breast feeding, teenagers, and young adults to age 24 need 3 servings.

Most of our clients eventually ask for a sample menu or guide to help them plan nutritious meals for themselves and their families. We have included menu guides for several calorie levels. These have been planned with the Dietary Guidelines for Americans in mind. We have added a few of our own guidelines and refer to the combination of both as FOUNDATION FOR FITNESS.

FOUNDATION FOR FITNESS

1. Consume at least 50-60 percent of your calories from carbohydrate containing foods such as grains, vegetables, fruits, low fat or skim milk products.

2. Increase fiber in your diet. This means more whole grain products, vegetables, fruits.

3. Eat less fat, saturated fat and cholesterol. This means more fish and poultry and choosing the leaner cuts of meat such as beef or pork. Reduce fat calories to 30 percent or less of total daily calorie intake.

4. Consume more fresh and minimally processed foods.

5. If you eat sugar-containing foods or alcohol, do so in moderation.

6. Eat at least three times a day. It is wise to avoid skipping meals. Recent evidence indicates snacks may be a positive habit.

7. Consume 1/2 to 2/3 of your day's intake before the evening meal.

8. Eat a variety of foods.

MENU GUIDES

The following menu guides will show you what meals with a high carbohydrate, low fat distribution of calories look like. The fat level is below 30 percent of calories and the carbohydrate level is above 50 percent of the calories. People who eat like this will be more nutritionally fit and will probably have less chance of developing heart disease. Please use these outlines only as a means of making more informed selections of calories. Please don't view them as another "diet" you have to follow.

SPECIAL NOTE FOR USING MENU GUIDES:

We have suggested eating certain foods such as 2 slices of whole wheat bread on the menu guides. However, there may be times when you don't want bread. When this happens, select other carbohydrate containing foods such as other cereal products or fruits or vegetables which have the same number of calorie points as the 2 slices of bread. We did not list the fat grams for these meals because individual food choices will have some bearing on the total fat grams. Most of the time the fat intake will be less than 30 percent of your calories. We chose to show 1400 and 1600 calorie levels because people usually do not realize that with low fat choices of food, there is quite a lot of food to eat.

MENU GUIDE FOR APPROXIMATELY 1400 CALORIES

BREAKFAST
*1 egg, prepared without fat or 1 ounce low fat or part skim milk cheese
2 slices whole wheat toast (can omit egg and add 1 additional slice toast)
1 cup skim milk
6 ounces of citrus fruit juice or vegetable juice or 1 piece of fresh fruit
1 teaspoon of margarine or 2 teaspoons of "diet" margarine

Total calorie points for breakfast = 5.5

LUNCH
2 ounces very lean meat, fish or poultry, prepared without fat or flour
1/2-1 cup green or yellow vegetables, prepared without fat
2 slices of whole wheat bread
1 piece of fresh fruit
2 teaspoons of margarine or mayonnaise or 4 teaspoons of "diet" margarine

Total calorie points for lunch = 5

SNACK
1 cup dry cereal or 3/4 cup cooked cereal or 1 1/2 slices bread
1 cup skim milk
1 piece fresh fruit

Total calorie points for snack = 3.5

DINNER
2 ounces of very lean meat, fish or poultry, prepared without fat or flour
1 large baked potato or 1 cup corn, beans, peas, pasta product or rice
1/2-1 cup green or yellow vegetables, prepared without fat
2 teaspoons of regular margarine or 4 teaspoon "diet" margarine

Total calorie points for dinner = 5

*To reduce cholesterol in the diet, you may want to limit egg yolks to no more than three-four per week.

MENU GUIDE FOR APPROXIMATELY 1600 CALORIES

BREAKFAST
*1 egg, prepared without fat or 1 ounce low fat or part skim milk cheese

2 slices whole wheat toast (can omit egg and add 1 additional slice toast)

1 cup skim milk

12 ounces of citrus fruit juice or vegetable juice or 2 pieces of fresh fruit

1 teaspoon of margarine or 2 teaspoons of "diet" margarine

Total calorie points for breakfast = 6.5

LUNCH
3 ounces very lean meat, fish or poultry, prepared without fat or flour

1/2-1 cup green or yellow vegetables, prepared without fat

2 slices of whole wheat bread

1 piece of fresh fruit

2 teaspoons of margarine or mayonnaise or 4 teaspoons of "diet' margarine

Total calorie points for lunch = 6.25

SNACK
1 cup dry cereal or 3/4 cup cooked cereal or 1 1/2 slices bread

1 cup skim milk

1 piece of fresh fruit

Total calorie points for snack = 3

DINNER
3 ounces very lean meat, fish or poultry, prepared without fat or flour

1 large baked potato or 1 cup corn, beans, pasta product or rice

1/2-1 cup green or yellow vegetables, prepared without fat

2 teaspoons regular margarine or 4 teaspoons "diet" margarine

Total calorie points for dinner 5.75

*To reduce cholesterol in the diet, you may want to limit egg yolks to no more than three–four per week.

NUTRITION QUALITY CHECK
We would recommend a nutrition quality check. This is a different type of food diary from the one presented earlier, which only asked for a count of fat, calorie, sodium, or fiber intake. Data collected on the diary sheet presented on the next page will give you an idea about whether or not you are consuming an adequate diet. Make a tally mark under each food grouping when you have eaten a serving of food listed there. Mixed dishes such as chili or spaghetti will be marked under more than one category of food. Continue for each meal for a week and total your tally marks for the entire week under the column labelled WEEKLY TOTALS. Compare your diet from week to week.

NUTRITION QUALITY CHECK

TYPE OF FOOD	NUMBER OF SERVINGS	WEEKLY TOTALS	WEEKLY GOALS
MILK PRODUCTS			14
1 Cup Skim Milk Or Yogurt	_____	_____	
1 1/2 Ounce of Cheese	_____	_____	
1 Cup Milk Base Pudding	_____	_____	
1 3/4 Cups Ice Cream	_____	_____	
2 Cups Cottage Cheese	_____	_____	
PROTEIN FOODS			14-21
2 Ounces Cooked Fish, Poultry, Meat	_____	_____	
2 Eggs	_____	_____	
1 Cup Cooked Dried Beans, Peas, Lentils	_____	_____	
5 Tablespoons Peanut Butter	_____	_____	
FRUITS-VEGETABLES			35+
1/2 Cup Cooked Or Juice	_____	_____	
1 Cup Raw	_____	_____	
1 Piece Fresh Fruit	_____	_____	
GRAIN GROUP			42+
1 Slice Whole Grain Bread	_____	_____	
1 Cup Cold Cereal, WG	_____	_____	
1/2 Cup Cooked Cereal, Pasta, Grits	_____	_____	
FAT POINTS	_____	_____	_____
ALCOHOLIC BEVERAGES	_____	_____	

For example, if you eat the following breakfast: 1 cup orange juice, 2 slices of whole wheat toast, 1 cup Wheaties, and 1 cup skim milk, your tally sheet would look something like this.

1 Cup Milk or Yogurt	I
1/2 Cup Juice	II
1 Slice Whole Grain Bread	II
1 Cup Cold Cereal, WG	I

A word to the wise, the foods listed above are not equal in either fat or calorie content. They are grouped together because they are approximately equal in other nutrient content such as vitamins, minerals, protein, etc.

Chapter 11

SALT, SALT EVERYWHERE AND NOTHING LEFT TO EAT

• Are you perplexed about what's left to eat when you've been told you can't have salt?

• Are you confused about the difference between salt and sodium?

• Are you fed up with foods that taste blah after you've shaken the salt habit?

• If you answered "yes" to any of the above questions, this section is just for you.

SALT IS IN EVERYTHING!

This is doubtless your impression if you've read many labels in the grocery store recently. Salt is the second most popular food additive in this country; sugar is first. Salt is composed of two minerals, sodium and chloride. Sodium, approximately 40 percent of salt, is the real culprit if you're trying to reduce salt in your diet. The sodium in foods is usually measured in milligrams. A milligram is 1/1000 of a gram. To put this into perspective, a gram is about the weight of a paper clip. Low sodium diets prescribed by physicians ordinarily are 2-3 grams of sodium a day. This means total food eaten during a day's time should contain no more than 2000 or 3000 milligrams of sodium.

One way of staying within the prescribed limit is to consult pamphlets which show the sodium content of foods and then to add up milligrams of sodium in each kind and amount of food eaten. For example, you would add 142 milligrams of sodium for a slice of bread, 36 milligrams of sodium for 3 ounces of rump roast prepared without salt, and 70 milligrams for two 8 inch stalks of celery, etc. This is tedious work for most of us.

POINTS ARE EASIER

As with calories, smaller numbers or units are less of a drag to add and to remember. Try adding 6 sodium points for a slice of bread, 2 for the roast beef and 3 for the celery stalk and you won't need a calculator.

Points work for sodium as well as for calories—here's how. One sodium point is approximately 23 milligrams of sodium. So your low sodium diet of 2000 or 3000 milligrams of sodium is equal to 87 or 130 sodium points for the day—a much more manageable sum. To convert other levels of sodium in the diet to points, consult the table on page 58.

HERE'S HOW YOU "CAN HAVE" SOME OF THOSE FOODS YOU NEVER THOUGHT YOU'D EAT AGAIN AND STILL LIMIT SODIUM INTAKE

We can't promise you a pickle binge, but you'll be surprised at what you "can have" and still be within safe sodium limits. You may have to ignore the lists of forbidden foods provided by most low sodium diets and be willing to engage in some creative choosing and a little arithmetic.

The ham you've longed for might still be yours! Salt cured ham is generally considered one of the most menacing foods in a low sodium diet. But, consider this: 1 ounce of lean ham is worth 17 points. Should you decide to eat 1 ounce of ham with your navy beans, this still leaves a reasonably generous 70 sodium points for the rest of the day if your total sodium points are 87. Even salt can be used with caution. A carefully measured level one-fourth teaspoon of salt will cost you about 25 sodium points. If you choose to work salt into your points, we would recommend putting the day's measured amount in your own private salt shaker. If you have some left over, it should **not** be added to the next day's ration. Discard any leftover salt and start fresh the next day.

READ ALL LABELS

Salt is not the only place where sodium occurs. A brief glance at any grocery shelf will reveal an abundance of other compounds containing sodium. It is wise to avoid eating any food which has any of the following ingredients added **unless** you know the number of sodium points for that particular food: salt, baking soda, baking powder, di-sodium phosphate, sodium alginate, sodium benzoate, sodium hydroxide, sodium proprionate, sodium sulfite, and monosodium glutamate.

NUTRIENT INSURANCE

Counting sodium points is important but there are about 40 other nutrients that count too. You could choose to spend all of your sodium budget for pickles, olives and corned beef, but this might not leave you enough to spare for all of the foods essential for good health. To insure an adequate intake of these nutrients, consume all the foods listed in the Nutrient Insurance Guide on page 46. You will find yourself eating more vegetables, fruits and whole grain or enriched breads and cereals to improve your odds of getting a nutritionally adequate diet. Fortunately, fresh or frozen fruits and vegetables without salt or sugar are nutritional giants as well as low sodium bargains.

SPECIAL NOTE FOR PEOPLE WITH HYPERTENSION (HIGH BLOOD PRESSURE)

Your sodium intake is not the whole story! Loss of body fat is helpful in controlling blood pressure. Many people who reduce their percentage of body fat by only a few pounds have been able to reduce their need for medication, and some have been able to eliminate their medication altogether. Exercise can be a big boon in body fat loss.

POTASSIUM

Some medicines that are prescribed for high blood pressure deplete the body of potassium, an essential mineral. Therefore, for some of you it may be necessary to eat a diet rich in potassium. However, you should consult your physician before increasing potassium in your diet since some types of kidney disease can cause too much potassium to build up in your system. Some salt substitutes are high in potassium. We recommend that you consult your physician before using these to season your foods. Fruits and vegetables and fluid milks or yogurt are excellent potassium sources. Actually, some studies suggest that a diet high in potassium and low in sodium is protective against high blood pressure.

CALCIUM AND MAGNESIUM

Recently, some authorities are stressing the importance of adequate intakes of calcium and magnesium in all of our diets, particularly for those people with high blood pressure. These three minerals, potassium, calcium, and magnesium, and their relationship to high blood pressure are areas of continuing research.

Foods high in calcium are dairy products (use skim milk to lower fat and cholesterol intake) and green leafy vegetables. Foods high in magnesium are dried peas and beans, nuts, whole grain cereals, cocoa, chocolate and green leafy vegetables.

It comes back to this: Mother was right, "Drink your milk, and eat your vegetables, fruits and whole grain cereals."

TABLE 11-1
HOW DO YOU CONVERT YOUR DAILY SODIUM LEVEL TO SODIUM POINTS?

If your physician has not set a sodium level, aim for between 2000 and 3000 milligrams of sodium (87 to 130 points) per day. Otherwise check the chart below for the level he/she has prescribed.

Daily Sodium Level (Milligrams)	Sodium Points for the Day	Daily Sodium Level (Milligrams)	Sodium Points for the Day
500	22	2000	87
1000	43	2500	109
1250	54	3000	130
1500	65	3500	152
1750	76		

SPECIAL NOTES:

The 1989 U.S. Recommended Dietary Allowances has set 500 milligrams of sodium per day as the minimum requirement.

MAKE INFORMED CHOICES.

Just as with the fat and calorie information, we hope you will use the sodium information to make informed choices of foods. Use generous amounts of herbs, spices and lemon juice to season foods. One client made up a basket of condiments he could sprinkle on at the table when he needed to add zip to something he was eating. The basket included garlic and onion powder, seasoned pepper, tabasco sauce, a plastic squeeze bottle of lemon juice, an herb and spice blend, plus dill weed and a few other of his favorite herbs. Let your imagination be your guide!

Chapter 12

PLANNING A DIET FOR PEOPLE WITH DIABETES USING FAT GRAMS AND CALORIE POINTS

The following guidelines are the backbone of healthy food choices for people with diabetes mellitus. You may notice few differences from the guidelines for good health which we have been discussing in previous chapters.

IF OVERFAT, READ THE CHAPTERS ON LOSING BODY FAT.
One of the best ways to decrease blood glucose (sugar) is to decrease body fat. Often, just a few pounds less of body fat can make a big difference. As with people who do not have diabetes, exercise is the bottom line. So, if you have an elevated blood sugar level and are overfat, consult your physician and dietitian or other diabetes educator before proceeding. The first part of this book can provide a good starter guide for you. We have a list of recommended readings in Appendix C on page 134 which will give you more information about diabetes than is possible in this small book.
If you have a calorie prescription from your doctor or dietitian, use the fat and calorie information in Chapter Seven and in the food tables. If you have diabetes, it is not a good idea to practice the averaging of calories, especially if you are taking insulin.

AVOID SKIPPING MEALS.
A minimum of three meals per day is recommended. You will probably find an afternoon and/or evening snack desirable. Discuss your best meal and snack distribution with a registered dietitian or other certified diabetes educator.
Learning to do home glucose monitoring will give you the needed information about when you need food and the effect certain foods or combinations of foods have on your blood sugar. In other words, you can be in control of your own food choices.

EAT MORE FIBER AND STARCH AND LESS FAT!
The good news is . . . your diet is composed of ordinary foods, just more of some and less of others. Research shows that a diet that is high in fiber, high in complex carbohydrates (50–60% of your calories), and low in fat helps control blood sugar and lowers cholesterol and triglycerides in the blood. People with diabetes have an increased risk of heart disease, so lowering blood levels of both cholesterol and triglycerides is highly desirable. Consult Chapter Nine beginning on page 36 for guidelines on lowering cholesterol and triglycerides.

A DIET TO CONTROL BLOOD GLUCOSE IS:

I. High in fiber. Increase fiber by:
   a. Eating fruits instead of the juice whenever possible.
   b. Eating whole wheat or bran bread or whole grain cereals instead of white bread or refined cereals.
   c. Eating a minimum of 1–2 servings of vegetables at each lunch and dinner.
   d. Including the amount of fiber which will assist in the control of blood sugar. See Appendix B on page 126 for a table of the fiber content of foods. Choose foods that will add up to at least 20 grams total fiber per 1000 calories per day and include at least 13–14 grams of soluble fiber in your total. You will want to increase fiber gradually in your diet.

II. Higher in complex carbohydrates (not sugar, honey, syrups, or foods containing these products). Foods which are high in sugar are marked with an **X** in the food tables. Complex carbohydrates are found in such foods as breads, potatoes, pasta products, crackers, dried beans, and cereal products (not presweetened). The type of fiber (soluble) found in dried beans, some cereals, fruits and vegetables seems especially beneficial in helping to reduce blood sugar. Some research indicates that the diet will work only if it contains a significant amount of fiber–containing foods.

III. Lower in total fat. Several things can be done to accomplish this:
   a. Keeping total fat grams below 35–50 per day if you are a woman or below 40–60 grams per day if you are a man. For more details on keeping fat below 20–30% of your calorie intake, read Chapter Seven.
   b. Limiting fish, poultry, and meat servings to 2–3 ounces at a meal.
   c. Consuming more fish and skinned poultry, rather than red meat. (Limit red meat to 3–5 servings per week.)
   d. Avoiding high fat meats such as luncheon meats, bacon, or sausage as often as possible.
   e. Eliminating fat in recipes or cutting down on amounts called for.
   f. Using lower fat salad dressings, lower calorie margarines, etc.
   g. Using skim milk instead of whole milk and lower fat cheeses instead of those with a higher fat content.
   h. Baking, broiling, and stewing, rather than frying. Sauté in dry white or red wines, bouillon or tomato juice instead of oils or other fats.
   i. Using low calorie pan sprays for frying.

REMEMBER, CONSULT CHAPTERS ONE THROUGH NINE FOR MORE INFORMATION ON FAT, FIBER AND CALORIES. FOR INFORMATION ON SODIUM, CONSULT CHAPTER ELEVEN . THE FOOD VALUE TABLES CONTAIN INFORMATION ON ALL THREE.

Chapter 13

HOW DO YOU CONVERT CALORIES AND SODIUM TO POINTS?

Although the food value tables in this book provide information on most commonly used foods, there are bound to be foods it was not possible to include. You can use the tables on the next two pages to convert calorie and sodium information into points.

For example, you have decided to eat a frozen dinner and that particular brand of frozen dinner is not included in the food value tables. Does this mean you cannot have this dinner? Not at all. Most foods have calories, fat and sodium information listed somewhere on the package. If not, the information can be obtained by writing to the manufacturer.

HOW DO YOU CONVERT CALORIES TO CALORIE POINTS?

Let's start with calorie information. Find the number of calories per serving on the package. Then, look under Calories on the CALORIE CONVERSION TABLE below. Opposite the range of calorie values on the CALORIE CONVERSION TABLE are listed the number of Calorie Points for each range.

In the case of your frozen dinner, it is listed on the package as containing 450 calories. The number 450 falls in the range of 426–462 on the calorie side of the CALORIE CONVERSION TABLE. Look opposite this range for the number of calorie points in that food. In this case, 450 calories equals 6 calorie points.

TABLE 13-1
CALORIE CONVERSION TABLE

Calories	Calorie Points	Calories	Calorie Points
0-18	0	389-425	5.5
19-55	0.5	426-462	6
56-92	1	463-499	6.5
93-129	1.5	500-537	7
130-166	2	538-574	7.5
167-203	2.5	575-611	8
204-240	3	612-648	8.5
241-277	3.5	649-685	9
278-314	4	686-723	9.5
315-351	4.5	724-760	10
352-388	5	761-797	10.5

One calorie point is approximately 75 calories.

HOW DO YOU CONVERT SODIUM MILLIGRAMS TO SODIUM POINTS?

The same way you converted calories to calorie points. Look at your frozen dinner package and find the number of milligrams of sodium listed on the package. In this case, the number is 1168 milligrams of sodium. Find the Milligrams of Sodium column on the SODIUM CONVERSION TABLE below and locate the appropriate range of milligrams. Look opposite the range and note that the number of sodium points is 51.

TABLE 13-2
SODIUM CONVERSION TABLE

Milligrams of Sodium	Sodium Points	Milligrams of Sodium	Sodium Points
0-11	0	633-655	28
12-34	1	656-678	29
35-57	2	679-701	30
58-80	3	702-724	31
81-103	4	725-747	32
104-126	5	748-770	33
127-149	6	771-793	34
150-172	7	794-816	35
173-195	8	817-839	36
196-218	9	840-862	37
219-241	10	863-885	38
242-264	11	886-908	39
265-287	12	909-931	40
288-310	13	932-954	41
311-333	14	955-977	42
334-356	15	978-1000	43
357-379	16	1001-1023	44
380-402	17	1024-1046	45
403-425	18	1047-1069	46
426-448	19	1070-1092	47
449-471	20	1093-1115	48
472-494	21	1116-1138	49
495-517	22	1139-1161	50
518-540	23	1162-1184	51
541-563	24	1185-1207	52
564-586	25	1208-1230	53
587-609	26	1231-1253	54
610-632	27	1254-1276	55

One sodium point is approximately 23 milligrams of sodium.

SYMBOLS USED IN THE TABLE OF FOOD VALUES

X FOODS WITH SIGNIFICANT AMOUNT OF ADDED SUGAR

?– PROBABLY CONTAINS SODIUM, BUT AMOUNT UNKNOWN

TABLE OF FOOD VALUES

FOOD	SERVING SIZE	FAT GRAMS	CALORIE POINTS	SODIUM POINTS
STARCHY FOODS: BREAD AND CEREAL PRODUCTS				
Breads:				
Bagel	1	1	2	9
Biscuit, Made From Mix				
With Milk	1 (2" x 1.25")	3	1	12
Biscuit, Canned, From				
Refrigerator Dough	1	3	1	15
Bread, Raisin	1 slice	1	1	4
Bread, White	1 slice	1	1	6
Bread, White, Unsalted	1 slice	1	1	0
Bread, Whole Wheat	1 slice	1	1	6
Bread, Whole Grain, Roman				
Meal	1 slice	1	1	5
Breadcrumbs, Dry	1/4 cup	1	1.5	8
Breadsticks, No Salt				
Coating	1 stick (8" x 0.75")	0	0.5	2
Bun, Hamburger	1 bun (1.5 ounce)	1	1.5	10
Bun, Hotdog	1 bun (1 ounce)	1	1	7
Cornbread, From Mix With				
Egg & Milk	1 piece (2.5" x 2.5" x 1.5")	6	2.5	11
Croissant	1 roll	6	1.5	6
English Muffin	1 muffin	1	2	16
Matzo	1 piece	0	1.5	0
X Muffin:				
Blueberry, From Mix	1 muffin	4	1.5	9
Bran Or Plain	1 muffin	4	1.5	8
Corn	1 muffin	5	1.5	4
Rolls:				
Brown & Serve	1 roll (2.5" x 2")	2	1	6
Crescent, Refrigerator,				
Pillsbury	2 rolls	11	2.5	20
Bulgur, Cooked	1 cup	0	2	0
Cereals, Ready-To-Eat: (Note: Cereals are marked with an **X** for every teaspoon of sugar they contain and with **x** for every 1/2 teaspoon.)				
General Mills:				
Cheerios	1 1/4 cups	2	1.5	13
X Crispy Wheat 'N Raisins	3/4 cup	1	1.5	6
XX Golden Grahams	3/4 cup	1	1.5	12
XX Honey Nut Cheerios	3/4 cup	1	1.5	11
x Kix	1 1/2 cups	0	1.5	11
x Total	1 cup	1	1.5	10
x Triples	3/4 cup	1	1.5	11
XXx Trix	1 cup	1	1.5	6
x Wheaties	1 cup	1	1.5	9
Kelloggs:				
X All-Bran	1/3 cup	1	1	11
X Bran Flakes	2/3 cup	0	1	10
XX Cocoa Krispies	3/4 cup	0	1.5	8

FOOD	SERVING SIZE	FAT GRAMS	CALORIE POINTS	SODIUM POINTS
Kelloggs:				
x Cornflakes	1 cup	0	1.5	13
XXx Corn Pops	1 cup	0	1.5	4
Xx Cracklin Oat Bran	1/2 cup	3	1.5	6
x Crispix	1 cup	0	1.5	10
X Frosted Mini-Wheats	4 biscuits	0	1.5	0
XXx Fruit Loops	1 cup	1	1.5	5
XX Just Right	3/4 cup	1	2	7
XX Lightly Frosted Bran	2/3 cup	0	1.5	8
XX Low Fat Granola	1/3 cup	2	1.5	3
Xx Mueslix, GoldenCrunch	1/2 cup	2	1.5	7
XX Nut & Honey Crunch	2/3 cup	1	1.5	9
x Rice Krispies	1 cup	0	1.5	13
Shredded Wheat:				
Spoon Size	2/3 cup	0	1	0
Biscuit	1	0	1	0
Malt-o-Meal:				
Puffed Wheat	1 cup	0	0.5	0
x Crisp 'N Crackling Rice	1 cup	0	1.5	10
Post's:				
XX Alpha-Bits	1 cup	1	1.5	8
XXx Cocoa Pebbles	3/4 cup	1	1.5	7
x Crispy Critters	1 cup	0	1.5	10
X Fruit & Fibre	2/3 cup	2	1.5	7
XXx Fruity Pebbles	3/4 cup	1	1.5	6
x Grapenuts	1/4 cup	0	1.5	7
X Grapenuts Flakes	7/8 cup	1	1.5	6
X Honey Bunches Of Oats	2/3 cup	2	1.5	8
XX Honeycomb	1 1/3 cups	0	1.5	8
x Post Toasties	1 1/4 cups	0	1.5	13
Xx Raisin Bran	2/3 cup	1	1.5	10
Quaker:				
XX Cap 'n Crunch's Peanut				
Butter Crunch	3/4 cup	3	1.5	10
X Life	2/3 cup	2	1.5	7
XX Honey & Raisins Cereal	1/4 cup	5	2	1
Ralston:				
x Corn Chex	1 cup	0	1.5	13
XX Cookie Crisp	1 cup	1	1.5	6
X Multi-Bran Chex	2/3 cup	1	1	9
X Muesli, Pecan Peach,				
Almond Raspberry Or				
Walnut Cranberry	1/2 cup	3	2	4
x Rice Chex	1 1/8 cups	0	1.5	10
x Wheat Chex	2/3 cup	1	1.5	10
Cereals, Cooked (Unless Specified Otherwise):				
Bulgur	1/2 cup	0	1	0
Corn Grits:				
Regular & Quick	1 cup	0	2	0

FOOD	SERVING SIZE	FAT GRAMS	CALORIE POINTS	SODIUM POINTS
Cereals, Cooked (Unless Specified Otherwise):				
Corn Grits:				
Instant, Plain	1 packet	0	1	15
Cream Of Rice	1/2 cup	0	1	0
Cream Of Wheat:				
Quick	1/2 cup	0	1	3 .
Instant	1/2 cup	0	1	0
Mix N' Eat:				
Plain	1 packet	0	1.5	10
X Flavored	1 packet	0	2	10
Farina, Without Salt	1/2 cup	0	2	0
Malt-O-Meal, Plain &				
Chocolate Products	1/2 cup	0	1	0
Oats:				
Oat Bran, Dry	1/3 cup	2	1	0
Regular, Quick &				
Instant	1/2 cup	1	1	0
Instant:				
Plain	1 packet	2	1.5	12
X Maple & Brown Sugar	1 packet	2	2	12
Ralston	1/2 cup	0	1	0
Chow Mein Noodles	1/2 cup	7	1.5	4
Cornmeal, Degermed	1/4 cup	1	1.5	0
Couscous	1/2 cup	0	1.5	0
Crackers:				
Butter Rounds	10 crackers	6	2	16
Cheese Rounds	10 crackers	7	2	16
Goldfish	12 crackers	2	0.5	2
Graham	2 squares	1	0.5	4
Harvest Crisps, Oat Or				
5-Grain	6 crackers	2	1	6
HiHo	4 crackers	5	1	?-
Melba Toast	2 crackers	0	0.5	0
Mini-Crispys Rice Cake Snacks				
Honey-Almond	2 cakes	0	0.5	1
Nutty Wheat Thins	7 crackers	4	1	7
Oat Thins	8 crackers	3	1	4
Oyster	36 crackers	2	1.5	12
Ritz Bits	22 crackers	4	1	5
Ritz Bits Peanut Butter				
Sandwiches	6 sandwiches	4	1	3
Cheese Ritz Bits	22 crackers	4	1	7
Ritz Or Ritz Cheese	4 crackers	5	1	6
Ryekrisp	3 triple crackers	0	1	6
Saltines Or Soda	10 crackers	3	1.5	14
Mild Cheddar, Sunshine	5 crackers	2	1	8
Sandwich Type:				
Cheese/Peanut Butter	6 sandwiches	10	3	18
Crackers/Cheese	6 sandwiches	9	2.5	26
Soda (Unsalted Tops)	10 crackers	3	1.5	9

FOOD	SERVING SIZE	FAT GRAMS	CALORIE POINTS	SODIUM POINTS
Crackers:				
Snack Wells:				
Cheese, Reduced Fat	18 crackers	1	1	7
Wheat, Fat Free	5 crackers	0	0.5	7
Triscuits	3 crackers	2	1	3
Vegetable Thins	7 crackers	4	1	6
Waverly Wafers	4 crackers	3	1	7
Wheat Thins	8 crackers	3	1	5
Zwieback	2 crackers	1	1	1
Flour:				
Rice, White	1/2 cup	1	4	0
Wheat, All Purpose	1/2 cup	1	3	0
Whole Wheat	1/2 cup	1	2.5	0
Hominy, Canned	1/2 cup	1	1	7
Pancake:				
Made From Mix				
With Egg & Milk	1 cake (6" x 0.5")	5	2	18
Frozen:				
Hungry Jack	3 cakes	4	3	25
Krusteaz, Blueberry	3 cakes	5	4	31
Pasta, Enriched, Unsalted Cooked Tender:				
Macaroni	1 cup	2	2	0
Noodles, Egg	1 cup	2	2.5	0
Spaghetti	1 cup	1	2	0
Rice, Unsalted, Cooked:				
Brown	1 cup	1	3	0
White	1 cup	0	3	0
Wild	1 cup	0	2	0
Rice Cake	1 cake	0	0.5	1
Stuffing:				
Bread, Mix Dry Form:				
Cubes	1 cup	2	2	18
Coarse Crumbs	1 cup	2	4	40
Cornbread, Stovetop	1 cup	18	5	50
Tapioca, Dry	1/4 cup	0	2	0
Tortilla, Corn	1 (6"diam.)	1	1	2
Waffle:				
Made From Mix With				
Egg & Milk	1 (7" x 0.5")	8	3	22
Nutri-Grain, Eggo, Frozen	2 waffles	10	3.5	26
Wheat Bran, Crude	1/4 cup	1	0.5	0
Wheat Germ, Toasted	1/4 cup	3	1.5	0

FRUITS AND FRUIT JUICES

FOOD	SERVING SIZE	FAT GRAMS	CALORIE POINTS	SODIUM POINTS
Apple:				
Raw With Skin	1 (3" diam. approx. 3/#)	1	1	0
Canned:				
Sauce, Unsweetened	1 cup	0	1.5	0
X Sauce, Sweetened	1 cup	1	2.5	0

FOOD	SERVING SIZE	FAT GRAMS	CALORIE POINTS	SODIUM POINTS
FRUITS AND FRUIT JUICES				
Apple:				
Dried, Uncooked	1/2 cup	0	1.5	2
Juice	1 cup	0	1.5	0
Apricots:				
Raw	3	0	0.5	0
Canned, Solids & Liquids:				
Water Pack	4	0	0.5	1
Juice Pack	3 halves	0	0.5	0
X Syrup Pack, Heavy	2	0	1	0
X Syrup Pack, Lite	3	0	0.5	0
Dried, Uncooked	10 medium halves	0	1	0
X Nectar, Canned	1 cup	0	2	0
Avocado	1/2 (3"diam.)	15	2	0
Banana	1 medium (9" long)	1	1.5	0
Blackberries	1 cup	1	1	0
Blueberries	1 cup	1	1	0
Cantaloupe	1/2 (5" diam.)	1	1.5	1
Cherries:				
Raw:				
Sour Red, Pitted	1 cup	1	1	0
Sweet	1 cup	1	1.5	0
Canned, Solids & Liquids:				
Water Pack:				
Sour Red, Pitted	1 cup	0	1	1
Sweet	1 cup	0	1.5	0
Sweet, Juice Pack	1 cup	0	2	0
X Sweet, Syrup Pack, Heavy	1 cup	0	3	0
Cranberries:				
Raw, Whole	1 cup	0	0.5	0
X Sauce, Canned, Sweetened	1/4 cup	0	1.5	1
X Cranberry Juice Cocktail, Sweetened	1 cup	0	2	0
Currants, Dried	1/4 cup	0	1.5	0
Dates	5	0	1.5	0
Figs:				
Raw	1 medium	0	0.5	0
Canned, Solids & Liquids,				
X Syrup Pack, Heavy	3 figs	0	1	0
Dried, Uncooked	1 (2"x1")	0	0.5	0
Fruit Cocktail:				
Canned, Solids & Liquids:				
Water Pack	1 cup	0	1	0
Juice Pack	1 cup	0	1.5	0
X Syrup Pack, Heavy	1 cup	0	2.5	1
Grapefruit:				
Raw	1/2 (4" diam.)	0	0.5	0

FOOD	SERVING SIZE	FAT GRAMS	CALORIE POINTS	SODIUM POINTS
FRUITS AND FRUIT JUICES				
Grapefruit:				
Sections, Canned, Solids & Liquids:				
Water Pack	1 cup	0	1	0
Juice Pack	1 cup	0	1.5	1
X Syrup Pack	1 cup	0	2	0
Juice, Canned				
Unsweetened	1 cup	0	1.5	0
Grapes:				
Raw:				
Slip Skin	1 cup	0	1	0
Seedless, Adherent				
Skin	1 cup	1	1.5	0
Canned, Solids & Liquids:				
Thompson Seedless,				
Water Pack	1 cup	0	1.5	1
X Syrup Pack, Heavy	1 cup	0	2.5	1
X Juice:				
Canned Or Bottled	1 cup	0	2	0
Frozen Concentrate,				
Diluted (3:1)	1 cup	0	1.5	0
Honeydew Melon	1 wedge (7" x 2")	0	0.5	1
Kiwifruit	1 medium	0	0.5	0
Lemon Or Lime Juice	1/2 cup	0	0.5	0
Mangos, Raw	1 cup slices	1	1.5	0
Nectarines	1 (2.5" diam.)	1	1	0
Oranges:				
Raw	1 (2.5" diam.)	0	1	0
Juice, Frozen Concentrate,				
Diluted (3:1)	1 cup	0	1.5	0
Papaya, Raw	1 fruit	0	1.5	0
Peaches:				
Raw	1 (2.5" diam.)	0	0.5	0
Canned, Halves Or Slices, Solids & Liquids:				
Juice Pack	1 cup	0	1.5	0
X Syrup Pack, Heavy	1 cup	0	2.5	0
Water Pack	1 cup	0	1	0
Dried, Uncooked	5 halves	1	2	0
X Frozen, Sliced,				
Sweetened	1/2 cup	0	1.5	0
X Nectar, Canned	1 cup	0	2	1
Pears:				
Raw, Bartletts	1 (2 .5" x 3.5")	1	1.5	0
Canned, Halves, Solids & Liquids:				
Juice Pack	1 cup	0	1.5	0
X Syrup Pack, Heavy	1 cup	0	2.5	1
Water Pack	1 cup	0	1	0
Dried, Uncooked	5 halves	1	3	0

FOOD	SERVING SIZE	FAT GRAMS	CALORIE POINTS	SODIUM POINTS
Pear:				
X Nectar, Canned	1 cup	0	2	0
Pineapple:				
Raw	1 cup diced	1	1	0
Canned, Solids & Liquids:				
Juice Pack	1 cup	0	2	0
X Syrup Pack	1 cup	0	2.5	0
Water Pack	1 cup	0	1	0
Juice, Canned	1 cup	0	2	0
Plantain, Cooked	1 cup sliced	0	2.5	0
Plums:				
Raw	1 (2" diam.)	0	0.5	0
Canned, Solids & Liquids:				
Juice Pack	3	0	0.5	0
X Syrup Pack, Heavy	3	0	1.5	1
Water Pack	3	0	0.5	0
Prunes:				
X Canned, Syrup Pack,				
Solids And Liquids	5	0	1	0
Dried, Uncooked	5	0	1.5	0
Juice, Canned	1 cup	0	2.5	0
Raisins, Seedless	1/4 cup	0	1.5	0
Raspberries:				
Raw	1 cup	1	1	0
X Frozen, Sweetened	1 cup	0	3.5	0
Rhubarb, Raw	1 cup diced	0	0.5	0
Strawberries:				
Raw	1 cup	1	0.5	0
X Frozen, Sliced,				
Sweetened	1 cup	0	3.5	0
Tangerines	1 (2 1/2" diam.)	0	0.5	0
Watermelon	1 slice (10"x1")	2	2	0

VEGETABLES, COOKED, WITHOUT FAT, SAUCES OR OTHER INGREDIENTS, UNLESS SPECIFIED OTHERWISE

FOOD	SERVING SIZE	FAT GRAMS	CALORIE POINTS	SODIUM POINTS
Arugula, Raw	1 cup	0	0	0
Alfalfa Sprouts, Raw	1 cup	0	1	0
Artichoke Hearts	1 cup	0	1	7
Artichoke Hearts, Frozen	1 (9 oz. box)	1	1.5	5
Asparagus:				
Spears	1 cup	1	0.5	1
Spears, Frozen	1 (10 oz. box)	1	1	1
Canned, Solids & Liquids	1 can	1	1	62
Bamboo Shoots	1 cup	1	0.5	0
Beans:				
Baked:				
Homemade	1 cup	13	5	46
Canned:				
Black	1 cup	1	3	40

FOOD	SERVING SIZE	FAT GRAMS	CALORIE POINTS	SODIUM POINTS
Beans:				
Canned:				
Chili, Mexican Style	1 cup	14	4	58
Cow-Peas/Crowder	1 cup	1	2.5	31
Garbanzo/Chickpeas	1 cup	3	4	31
Kidney	1 cup	1	3	39
Navy	1 cup	1	4	51
Pinto	1 cup	1	2.5	43
Plain Or Vegetarian	1 cup	1	3	44
Pork/Tomato Sauce	1 cup	2	3.5	48
Refried	1 cup	3	3.5	47
Snap, (Italian, Green Or Yellow)	1 can, drained	0	0.5	29
Three Bean Salad	1 cup	0	2.5	48
With Franks	1 cup	17	5	48
Dry, Most Varieties	1 cup	1	3	0
Hummus, Homemade	1 cup	21	5.5	26
Lentils, Boiled	1 cup	1	3	0
Lima:				
Fresh	1 cup	1	3	0
Baby, Frozen	1 (10 oz. box)	1	4.5	4
Fordhook, Frozen	1 (10 oz. box)	1	4	7
Mung Sprouts, Raw	1 cup	0	0.5	0
Snap (Italian, Green Or Yellow)	1 cup	0	0.5	0
Soybeans And Soybean Products:				
Boiled, Plain	1 cup	12	4	0
Roasted, Dry	1 cup	37	10.5	0
Miso	1/2 cup	8	4	219
Natto	1/2 cup	10	2.5	0
Soy Milk	1 cup	5	1	1
Soy Sauce (Tamari)	1 tablespoon	0	0	44
Tempeh	1/2 cup	6	2	0
Tofu (Soybean Curd):				
Raw, Firm	1/2 cup	11	2	1
Raw, Regular	1/2 cup	6	1.5	0
Beets:				
Sliced	1 cup	0	0.5	4
Canned, Solids & Liquids	1 cup	0	1	28
Harvard, Canned, Solids & Liquids	1 cup	0	2.5	17
Pickled, Sliced	1 cup	0	2	26
Greens	1 cup	0	0.5	15
Broccoli:				
Raw Or Cooked	1 spear	0	0.5	2
Frozen, Plain, Chopped	1 (10 oz. box)	1	1	2
Frozen, Cheese Sauce	1/2 cup	6	2	29
Brussels Sprouts:				
Fresh Or Frozen	1 cup	1	1	2
Frozen, Cheese Sauce	1/2 cup	6	2	24

FOOD	SERVING SIZE	FAT GRAMS	CALORIE POINTS	SODIUM POINTS
Cabbage:				
Cooked	1 cup	0	0.5	1
Raw	1 cup	0	0	1
Chinese, Raw	1 cup	0	0	2
Chinese, Cooked	1 cup	0	0.5	2
Coleslaw, Homemade Cream Style Dressing	1 cup	3	1	1
Carrots:				
Baby, Raw	10 carrots (approx. 3")	0	0.5	2
Carrot Raisin Salad, Homemade	1/2 cup	5	2	?–
Cooked, Drained	1 cup	0	1	5
Juice, Canned	1 cup	0	1.5	3
Raw	1	0	0.5	1
Cauliflower:				
Cooked Or Raw	1 cup	0	0.5	1
Frozen, Cheese Sauce	1/2 cup	6	1.5	21
Celery:				
Raw, Diced	1 cup	0	0.5	5
Stalk, Raw	4	0	0.5	6
Cooked, Diced	1 cup	0	0.5	6
Chard, Swiss, Chopped	1 cup	0	0.5	14
Chives	Any amount	0	0	0
Collards, Chopped	1 cup	0	0.5	1
Corn:				
Kernels	1 cup or 1 ear	2	2.5	1
Canned:				
Plain, Solids & Liquids	1 cup	1	2	28
Cream Style	1 cup	1	2.5	32
Hominy, White	1 cup	1	2	31
Cucumber, Raw	1	0	0.5	0
Dandelion Greens, Chopped	1 cup	1	0.5	2
Eggplant, Cubed	1 cup	0	0.5	0
Endive, Raw, Chopped	1 cup	0	0	1
Jerusalem Artichokes, Raw, Sliced	1 cup	0	1.5	?–
Kale, Cooked Or Raw, Chopped	1 cup	0	0.5	1
Kohlrabi	1 cup	0	0.5	1
Leek, Raw	1	0	1	1
Lettuce, Raw:				
Boston & Bibb Types	2 heads	1	0.5	1
Iceberg	1 head	1	1	2
Looseleaf, Shredded	1 cup (limit)	0	0	0
Romaine, Shredded	2 cups (limit)	0	0	0
Mushrooms:				
Canned, Drained	1 cup	0	0.5	52
Cooked, Drained	1 cup	1	0.5	0
Raw	1 cup pieces	0	0	0

FOOD	SERVING SIZE	FAT GRAMS	CALORIE POINTS	SODIUM POINTS
Mushrooms:				
Shiitake, Dried, Cooked	4 mushrooms	0	0.5	0
Mustard Greens, Chopped	1 cup	0	0.5	1
Mustard Greens, Frozen	1 (10 oz. box)	1	0.5	2
New Zealand Spinach, Chopped	1 cup	0	0.5	8
Okra, Fresh Or Frozen	8 pods	0	0.5	0
Onions:				
Cooked/Raw, Chopped	1/2 cup	0	0.5	0
Rings, Frozen, Prepared In Oven	7 rings	19	4	11
Canned, Solids & Liquids	1/2 cup	0	0.5	18
Green, Raw	2 medium (limit)	0	0	0
Parsley, Raw, Chopped	1 cup	0	0.5	1
Parsnips	1 cup	0	1.5	1
Peas:				
Edible-Pods, Cooked/Raw	1 cup	0	1	0
Edible-Pods, Frozen	1 (10 oz. box)	1	2	1
Green	1 cup	0	2	0
Green, Canned, Drained	1 can	1	3	30
Green, Frozen	1 (10 oz. box)	1	2.5	10
Green & Carrots, Canned	1 cup	1	1.5	29
Green & Carrots, Frozen	1 (10 oz. box)	1	2	8
Green & Onions, Frozen	1 cup	0	1	?–
Peppers:				
Green Or Red, Canned, Solids & Liquids	1 cup halves	0	0.5	83
Green, Red, Or Yellow Raw, Chopped	1 cup	0	0.5	0
Hot Chili, Canned, Solids & Liquids	1 cup	0	0.5	?–
Poi	1 cup	0	3.5	1
Potatoes:				
Au Gratin, Homemade	1 cup	19	4.5	46
Au Gratin, From Dry Mix	1 (5.5 oz. pkg.)	34	10.5	157
Baked With Skin	1 large	0	3	1
Boiled With Skin	1 medium	0	1.5	0
Canned, Solids & Liquids	1 can (1#)	1	2.5	59
Chips	1 ounce	10	2	6
From Dehydrated Flakes, With Milk & Salt	1 cup	12	3	30
French-Fried, Heated In Oven, Home	10 strips	4	1.5	1
Fried In Oil, Restaurant	10 strips	8	2	5
Hashed Brown, With Fat	1 cup	22	4	2
Mashed With Whole Milk & Fat, Salt Added	1 cup	5	2	21
Scalloped, Homemade	1 cup	9	3	36
Scalloped, From Dry Mix	1 (5.5 oz. pkg.)	35	10.5	122
Salad	1 cup	21	5	58

FOOD	SERVING SIZE	FAT GRAMS	CALORIE POINTS	SODIUM POINTS
Potatoes:				
Sticks	1 ounce	10	2	3
Sweet, Baked With Skin	1/2 cup	0	1.5	0
X Sweet, Canned, Syrup Pack, Solids & Liquids	1 cup	0	2.5	4
Tater Tots, Ore Ida	3 ounces	7	2	15
Pumpkin, Canned	1 cup	1	1	1
Radicchio, Shredded	1 cup	0	0	0
Radishes, Raw	10	0	0	0
Rhubarb, Frozen, Raw	1 cup	0	0.5	0
Rutabagas, Mashed	1 cup	0	1	1
Sauerkraut, Canned, Solids & Liquids	1 cup	0	0.5	68
Spinach:				
Canned, Solids & Liquids	1 cup	1	0.5	32
Cooked, Drained	1 cup	0	0.5	7
Frozen	1 (10 oz. box)	0	1	9
Raw, Chopped	1 cup	0	0	2
Souffle, Homemade	1 cup	18	3	33
Squash:				
Summer, Sliced, Cooked Or Raw	1 cup	0	0.5	0
Winter, Baked, Cubed	1 cup	1	1	0
Tomatoes:				
Green, Raw	1 medium	0	0.5	1
Canned:				
Juice	1 cup	0	0.5	19
Paste, Unsalted	1 cup	2	3	7
Tomatoes:				
Canned:				
Pureed, Salted	1 cup	0	1.5	43
Red, Ripe, Whole	1 cup	1	0.5	17
Sauce, Salted	1 cup	0	1	64
Red, Ripe, Raw	1 medium	0	0.5	0
Red, Ripe	1 cup pieces	1	1	1
Stewed, Homemade	1 cup	1	1	20
Sun-Dried	8 pieces	0	0.5	15
Spaghetti Sauce, Canned:				
Hunt's Traditional	1 cup	4	2	46
Prego, Extra Chunky	1 cup	10	3.5	55
Ragu, Chunky Garden Style	1 cup	6	2	38
Ragu, Natural	1 cup	8	2	64
Turnips:				
Cooked Or Raw, Cubed	1 cup	0	0.5	3
Greens, Chopped	1 cup	0	0.5	2
Greens, Canned, Solids & Liquids	1 can	1	1	51

FOOD	SERVING SIZE	FAT GRAMS	CALORIE POINTS	SODIUM POINTS
Vegetable Juice Cocktail	1 cup	0	0.5	38
Vegetables, Mixed:				
Canned, Drained	1 cup	0	1	24
Frozen	1 (10 oz. box)	1	2	4
Waterchestnuts, Canned,				
Solids & Liquids, Sliced	1/2 cup	0	0.5	0
Watercress, Raw	Any Amount	0	0	0

DAIRY PRODUCTS

FOOD	SERVING SIZE	FAT GRAMS	CALORIE POINTS	SODIUM POINTS
Cheeses:				
American Pasteurized				
Process Cheese	1 ounce	9	1.5	18
American, Kraft Free	1 ounce	0	0.5	19
American, Low-Fat	1 ounce	4	1	18
Blue	1 ounce	8	1.5	17
Cheddar	1 ounce	9	1.5	8
Colby	1 ounce	9	1.5	7
Cottage Cheese:				
Creamed	1/2 cup	5	1.5	20
2% Fat	1/2 cup	2	1.5	20
1% Fat	1/2 cup	1	1	20
Cream Cheese	2 tablespoons	10	1.5	4
Kraft Philadelphia Free	2 tablespoons	0	0.5	7
Edam	1 ounce	8	1.5	12
Feta	1 ounce	6	1	14
Free N' Lean, Alpine Lace	1 ounce	0	0.5	11
Goat, Semi-Soft	1 ounce	8	1.5	6
Goat, Soft	1 ounce	6	1	5
Gouda	1 ounce	8	1.5	10
Light 'N Lively Singles,				
Kraft	1 ounce	4	1	18
Monterey	1 ounce	9	1.5	7
Mozzarella, Low Moisture				
Part Skim Milk	1 ounce	5	1	7
Muenster	1 ounce	9	1.5	8
Neufchatel	1 ounce	7	1	5
Parmesan, Grated	2 tablespoons	3	0.5	8
Provolone	1 ounce	8	1.5	11
Ricotta, Part Skim Milk	1/2 cup	10	2.5	7
Romano	1 ounce	8	1.5	15
Roquefort	1 ounce	9	1.5	22
Swiss:				
Natural	1 ounce	9	1.5	3
Pasteurized Process	1 ounce	7	1.5	17
Cream:				
Half 'N Half	2 tablespoons	3	0.5	1
Sour	2 tablespoons	5	0.5	1
Whipping, Heavy, Fluid	1 tablespoon	6	0.5	0

FOOD	SERVING SIZE	FAT GRAMS	CALORIE POINTS	SODIUM POINTS
Cream Substitute:				
Frozen, Liquid	2 tablespoons	3	0.5	1
Powdered	1 tablespoon	3	0.5	1
Milk:				
Buttermilk, Cultured	1 cup	2	1.5	11
X Chocolate:				
Whole	1 cup	8	3	6
2% Fat	1 cup	5	2.5	7
1% Fat	1 cup	3	2	7
Canned:				
X Condensed, Sweet	1 cup	27	13	17
Evaporated Skim	1/2 cup	0	1.5	6
Evaporated Whole	1/2 cup	10	2.5	6
Dry, Nonfat, Instant	1/3 cup	0	1	5
Lowfat, 2%	1 cup	5	1.5	5
Lowfat, 1%	1 cup	3	1.5	5
Skim, With Nonfat Milk				
Solids Added	1 cup	1	1	6
Whole, 3.3% Fat	1 cup	8	2	5
Malted Milk Powder, Natural	1 tablespoon	2	1	4
X Milkshake	11 ounces	10	4.5	13
Yogurt, Lowfat:				
X Coffee And Vanilla	8 ounces	3	2.5	6
X Fruit Flavors	8 ounces	3	3	6
Yogurt, Plain, Non Fat	8 ounces	0	1.5	8

PROTEIN FOODS: MEAT, FISH, POULTRY AND EGGS

FOOD	SERVING SIZE	FAT GRAMS	CALORIE POINTS	SODIUM POINTS
Beef, Cooked:				
Breakfast Strips	3 strips	12	1.5	33
Brisket, Braised:				
Corned Beef	2 ounces	11	2	28
Flat, Fat & Lean	2 ounces	16	3	1
Flat, Lean Only	2 ounces	5	1.5	2
Point Half, Lean Only	2 ounces	9	2	2
Chuck, Pot Roast:				
Arm, Lean Only	2 ounces	4	1.5	2
Blade, Lean Only	2 ounces	10	2	2
Dried, Chipped	1 ounce	1	0.5	43
Flank Steak	2 ounces	7	2	2
Ground:				
Extra Lean, Healthy				
Choice	2 ounces	2	1	5
7% Fat With				
Carrageenan	2 ounces	5	1.5	2
Extra Lean & Lean				
(17-20% Fat)	2 ounces	9	2	2
Regular (27% Fat)	2 ounces	12	2	2
Rib:				
Roast, Fat & Lean	2 ounces	17	3	2
Roast, Lean Only	2 ounces	8	2	2

FOOD	SERVING SIZE	FAT GRAMS	CALORIE POINTS	SODIUM POINTS
Beef, Cooked:				
Rib:				
Steak, Fat & Lean	2 ounces	19	3	1
Steak, Lean Only	2 ounces	8	2	2
Short Ribs, Fat & Lean	2 ounces	24	3.5	1
Steaks, Lean & Fat:				
Porterhouse, Broiled	2 ounces	12	2.5	1
T-Bone, Broiled	2 ounces	14	2.5	1
Steaks, Lean Only:				
Porterhouse/T-Bone	2 ounces	6	1.5	2
Round Steak, Lean Only	2 ounces	4	1.5	2
Tenderloin, Lean & Fat:				
Broiled	2 ounces	10	2	1
Roasted	2 ounces	13	2.5	1
Tenderloin, Lean Only:				
Broiled	2 ounces	5	1.5	2
Roasted	2 ounces	6	1.5	1
Beefalo, Raw, Composite Cuts	4 ounces	5	2	4
Bison, Roasted	2 ounces	1	1	1
Deer, Roasted	2 ounces	1	2	1
Egg:				
Poached Or Boiled:				
Whole	1 large	5	1	3
White	2	0	0.5	5
Fried	1 large	7	1	7
Substitutes:				
Egg Beaters	1/4 cup	0	0.5	3
Healthy Choice	1/4 cup	0	0.5	4
Scramblers	1/4 cup	3	1	6
Fish:				
Anchovies, Canned In Oil, Drained	5 anchovies	2	0.5	32
Bass, Freshwater, Baked	3 ounces	4	1.5	3
Bass, Ocean, Baked	3 ounces	2	1.5	3
Bluefish, Baked	3 ounces	5	2	3
Clams, Canned, Drained	1/2 cup	1	1	3
Carp, Baked	3 ounces	6	2	2
Catfish, Channel, Breaded, Fried	3 ounces	11	2.5	10
Caviar, Black & Red	1 tablespoon	3	0.5	10
Cod, Broiled	3 ounces	1	1	3
Cod, Dried, Salted	3 ounces	2	3.5	260
Croaker, Breaded, Fried	3 ounces	11	2.5	13
Dolphinfish, Broiled	3 ounces	1	1.5	4
Eel, Baked	3 ounces	13	2.5	2

FOOD	SERVING SIZE	FAT GRAMS	CALORIE POINTS	SODIUM POINTS
Fish:				
Fish Cakes, Fillets, Sticks, Frozen, Breaded, Fried	3 ounces	10	3	21
Flounder Or Sole	3 ounces	1	1.5	4
Gefilte Fish, Canned	2 pieces	1	1	19
Grouper, Baked	3 ounces	1	1.5	2
Haddock, Broiled	3 ounces	1	1.5	3
Halibut, Baked	3 ounces	15	2.5	4
Herring:				
Baked	3 ounces	15	3	4
Kippered	1.5 ounces	5	1	16
Pickled	1 ounce	5	1	11
Mackerel:				
Broiled	3 ounces	9	2.5	4
Canned, Drained	1 can (#300)	23	7.5	59
Perch (Redfish), Broiled	3 ounces	1	1.5	3
Pike, Northern Or Walleye, Baked	3 ounces	1	1.5	2
Pollock, Baked	3 ounces	1	1.5	4
Pompano, Baked	3 ounces	10	2.5	3
Roughy, Orange, Baked	3 ounces	1	1	3
Salmon, Mixed Species:				
Broiled Or Baked	3 ounces	7	2	2
Canned, Pink With Bone	3 ounces	5	1.5	20
Smoked	3 ounces	4	1.5	29
Sardines, Canned, Drained	2 sardines	3	0.5	5
Seabass, Baked	3 ounces	2	1.5	3
Shark, Batter-Dipped, Fried	3 ounces	12	2.5	4
Snapper, Baked	3 ounces	2	1.5	2
Sturgeon, Baked	3 ounces	4	1.5	?-
Surimi	3 ounces	1	1	5
Swordfish, Baked	3 ounces	4	2	4
Trout, Mixed Species, Cooked	3 ounces	7	2	2
Tuna:				
Canned, Drained:				
In Oil	1 can (6.5 oz.)	14	4.5	26
In Water	1 can (6.5 oz.)	1	2.5	24
In Water, Low Sodium	1 can (6.5 oz.)	1	2.5	4
Broiled	3 ounces	1	1.5	2
Salad	1/2 cup	19	5	36
Turbot, Broiled	3 ounces	3	1.5	7
Whitefish, Cooked	3 ounces	6	2	2
Whiting, Baked	3 ounces	1	1.5	5
Shellfish:				
Crab:				
Canned, Drained	3 ounces	1	1	12

FOOD	SERVING SIZE	FAT GRAMS	CALORIE POINTS	SODIUM POINTS
Fish:				
Shellfish:				
Crab:				
Cakes, Fried	2 ounces	10	2	21
Dungeness,				
Steamed	3 ounces	1	1.5	14
Imitation	3 ounces	1	1	31
Soft Shell, Fried	1 crab (4.5 oz.)	18	4.5	49
Crayfish, Raw	3 ounces	0	1	1
Lobster, Boiled	3 ounces	2	1.5	8
Shrimp:				
Boiled	3 ounces	1	1	8
Breaded, Fried	3 ounces	10	3	13
Canned	3 ounces	2	1.5	6
Imitation	3 ounces	1	1.5	26
Mollusks:				
Abalone, Raw	3 ounces	1	1	14
Clams:				
Breaded, Fried	3 ounces	10	2.5	13
Canned, Drained	3 ounces	2	1.5	?–
Steamed	3 ounces	2	2	4
Mussels, Raw	3 ounces	2	1	11
Octopus, Cooked	3 ounces	2	2	?–
Oysters:				
Breaded, Fried	6 oysters	18	5	29
Canned	3 ounces	2	1	?–
Raw	3 oysters	3	1.5	7
Steamed	3 ounces	3	2	8
Scallops:				
Breaded, Fried	2 large	3	1	6
Imitation	3 ounces	0	1	29
Raw	3 ounces	1	1	6
Squid, Fried	3 ounces	6	2	11
Lamb, Lean:				
Arm And Blade:				
Lean & Fat	3 ounces	22	4	2
Lean Only	3 ounces	13	3.5	2
Leg, Lean Only	2 ounces	4	1.5	2
Loin Chop, Lean Only,				
Broiled	2 ounces	6	1.5	2
Luncheon Meats: See Sausages And Luncheon Meats				
Organ Meats:				
Heart, Beef, Braised	2 ounces	3	1.5	2
Kidney, Beef, Braised	2 ounces	2	1	3
Liver:				
Beef, Fried	2 ounces	5	1.5	3
Chicken, Simmered	2 ounces	3	1	1
Peanut Butter, Added Salt	2 tablespoons	16	2.5	7

FOOD	SERVING SIZE	FAT GRAMS	CALORIE POINTS	SODIUM POINTS
Pork, Fresh, Uncured:				
Center Loin Chop, Fried:				
Lean & Fat	2 ounces	17	3	2
Lean Only	2 ounces	9	2	2
Shoulder, Roasted:				
Lean & Fat	2 ounces	15	2.5	2
Lean Only	2 ounces	9	2	2
Spareribs, Lean & Fat, Braised	2 ounces	17	3	2
Tenderloin, Lean Only, Roasted	2 ounces	7	2	2
Pork Products, Cured:				
Bacon, Cooked	2 slices	6	1	9
Canadian Bacon, Grilled	2 ounces	5	1.5	38
Ham:				
Center Slice, Lean & Fat	2 ounces	7	1.5	34
Canned, Chopped	2 ounces	17	2.5	32
5% Fat	2 ounces	3	1	35
11% Fat	2 ounces	6	1.5	33
Salt Pork, Raw	1 ounce	23	3	18
Poultry:				
Chicken, Broilers/Fryers:				
Breast, Meat & Skin:				
Fried, With Flour	1/2 breast	9	3	3
Roasted	1/2 breast	8	2.5	3
Breast, Meat Only, Roasted	1/2 breast	3	2	3
Drumstick, Meat & Skin:				
Fried, With Flour	1 drumstick	7	1.5	2
Roasted	1 drumstick	6	1.5	2
Drumstick, Meat Only, Roasted	1 drumstick	3	1	2
Thigh, Meat & Skin:				
Fried, With Flour	1 thigh	9	2	2
Roasted	1 thigh	10	2	2
Thigh, Meat Only, Roasted	1 thigh	6	1.5	2
Wing, Meat & Skin, Fried, With Flour	1 wing	7	1.5	1
Wing, Meat Only, Roasted	1 wing	2	0.5	1
Duck, Domestic, Meat Only, Roasted	2 ounces	6	1.5	2
Goose, Domestic, Meat Only, Roasted	2 ounces	7	2	2
Turkey:				
Ground, Cooked	2 ounces	8	1.5	2

FOOD	SERVING SIZE	FAT GRAMS	CALORIE POINTS	SODIUM POINTS
Turkey:				
Roasted, With Skin:				
Light Meat	2 ounces	5	1.5	2
Dark Meat	2 ounces	7	1.5	2
Roasted Without Skin:				
Light Meat	2 ounces	2	1	2
Dark Meat	2 ounces	4	1.5	2
Poultry Food Products:				
Chicken, Canned, Boned, With Broth	1 can (5 oz.)	11	3	31
Turkey Bacon	1 slice	2	0.5	?–
Turkey Ham	2 ounces	3	1	25
Rabbit, Cooked, Composite Cuts	3 ounces	7	2.5	2
Sausages And Luncheon Meats:				
Bologna:				
97% Fat Free, Healthy Choice	1 ounce	1	0.5	12
Field Lite	1 ounce	6	1	13
Beef	1 ounce	8	1	12
Beef & Pork	1 ounce	10	1	13
Pork	1 ounce	6	1	15
Turkey	1 ounce	5	1	11
Bratwurst, Pork	1 link	22	3.5	21
Braunschweiger	2 ounces	16	3	28
Frankfurter:				
Beef	1 frank	16	2	20
Beef & Pork	1 frank	13	2	22
Chicken	1 frank	9	1.5	27
Jumbo Franks, Healthy Choice	1 frank	2	1	25
Light & Lean, Hormel	2 franks	2	1	30
Turkey, Louis Rich	1 frank	8	1.5	23
Turkey	1 frank	8	1.5	28
Liverwurst	2 ounces	16	2.5	?–
Pastrami, Turkey	2 ounces	4	1	26
Pepperoni	1 ounce (5 slices)	12	2	24
Sausage:				
Italian, Pork	1 link (5/#)	17	3	27
Polish	1 ounce	8	1	11
Pork	1 ounce or 2 links	8	2	21
Pork & Beef	1 ounce or 2 links	10	1.5	13
Salami:				
Beef And Pork	1 ounce	6	1	13
Turkey	2 ounces	7	1.5	25
Simulated Meat Products:				
Bacon	2 strips	5	0.5	10
Sausage	1 patty	7	1.5	15
Veal, Roasted	2 ounces	8	1.5	2

FOOD	SERVING SIZE	FAT GRAMS	CALORIE POINTS	SODIUM POINTS
FATS, OILS AND SALAD DRESSINGS				
Butter:				
Salted	1 teaspoon	4	0.5	2
Unsalted	1 teaspoon	4	0.5	0
Lard	1 tablespoon	13	1.5	0
Margarine:				
Salted	1 teaspoon	4	0.5	2
Unsalted	1 teaspoon	4	0.5	0
Liquid, Bottle	1 teaspoon	4	0.5	2
Low Calorie	2 teaspoons	4	0.5	1
Oil, Vegetable	1 tablespoon	14	1.5	0
Salad Dressing, Commercial:				
Blue Cheese	1 tablespoon	8	1	?–
French:				
Low Calorie	1 tablespoon	1	0.5	6
Regular	1 tablespoon	6	1	9
Hidden Valley Ranch, Buttermilk	1 tablespoon	3	1	5
Italian:				
Low Calorie	1 tablespoon	2	0	5
Regular	1 tablespoon	7	1	5
Mayonnaise	1 tablespoon	11	1.5	3
Mayonnaise Type:				
Regular	1 tablespoon	5	1	5
Fat Free	2 tablespoons	0	0.5	1
Russian:				
Low Calorie	1 tablespoon	1	0.5	6
Regular	1 tablespoon	8	1	6
Thousand Island:				
Low Calorie	1 tablespoon	2	0.5	7
Regular	1 tablespoon	6	1	5
Sandwich Spread, Commercial	1 tablespoon	5	1	?–
Shortening, Vegetable Oil, Hydrogenated	1 tablespoon	13	1.5	?–
DESSERTS AND SWEETS				
XCakes Baked From Mixes:				
Angelfood, No Icing	1/16 cake	0	1.5	3
DeLights, Duncan Hines, No Icing:				
Devil's Food	1/12 cake	5	2.5	15
Yellow	1/12 cake	4	2.5	12
Devil's Food With Chocolate Icing	1/12 cake	11	4	10
Gingerbread, No Icing	1 piece (3" x 3" x 1.5")	4	2.5	8

FOOD	SERVING SIZE	FAT GRAMS	CALORIE POINTS	SODIUM POINTS
XCakes Baked From Mixes:				
Lovin' Lites, Pillsbury, No Icing, Devil's Food Or Yellow	1/12 cake	3	2.5	17
Plain, No Icing	1 cupcake	4	1.5	6
Sugar Moist, Light, Betty Crocker, No Icing:				
Devil's Food	1/12 cake	4	2.5	16
Yellow	1/12 cake	4	2.5	13
White, Chocolate Icing	1/12 cake	10	4.5	9
Yellow, Chocolate Icing	1/12 cake	10	4	9
XCake Icing From Mix Or Ready To Spread	Amount for 1/12cake	7	2.5	4
XCandy:				
Caramels, Plain & Chocolate	1 ounce	3	1.5	3
Chocolate Chips, Semi-Sweet	1 cup	61	11.5	0
Fudge, Plain	1 ounce	4	1.5	2
Gum Drops, Hard, Jelly Beans	1 ounce	0	1.5	0
Life Savers	5 pieces	0	0.5	0
Marshmallow, Plain	3 large	0	1	0
Milk Chocolate, Plain	1 ounce	9	2	
With Peanuts	1 ounce	11	2	1
Peanut Brittle, No Salt Or Soda Added	1 ounce	3	1.5	0
XCheesecake, Frozen	1/6 cake	11	3	7
XCookies:				
Brownie With Nuts From Mix	1 (3" x 1" x 1")	4	1	1
Chocolate Chip, Homemade	2 (2.5")	6	1.5	3
Oatmeal With Raisins, Commercial	2 (2.5")	4	1.5	2
Sandwich Type, Chocolate Or Vanilla	2 (1.75")	5	1.5	4
Vanilla Wafers	5 (1.5")	2	1	2
XCustard, Baked From Mix	1/2 cup	5	2	10
XDessert Toppings:				
Butterscotch	3 tablespoons	0	2	5
Caramel	3 tablespoons	0	2	7
Chocolate Syrup	3 tablespoons	1	2	1
Strawberry	3 tablespoons	0	2	1
XWhipped Topping:				
Powdered, Prepared	1/4 cup	2	0.5	1
Semisolid, Frozen	1/4 cup	4	0.5	0
XDoughnut, Plain:				
Cake Type	1 (3.25" x 1")	8	2	9
Yeast Leavened	1 (3.75" x 1")	11	2.5	4

FOOD	SERVING SIZE	FAT GRAMS	CALORIE POINTS	SODIUM POINTS
XGelatin Dessert, Plain	1/2 cup	0	1	3
XGelatin Dessert With Fruit	1/2 cup	0	1	2
XGranola Bar	1 bar	4	1.5	3
XHoney	1 tablespoon	0	1	0
XIce Cream, 10% Fat	1/2 cup	7	2	3
XIce Cream Cone, No Ice Cream	1 cone	0	0.5	1
XIce Milk, Vanilla:				
Hardened	1/2 cup	3	1	2
Soft Serve	1/2 cup	12	1.5	4
XJams, Jellies, & Preserves	2 tablespoons	0	1.5	0
Pie Crust, Baked	1 shell	60	12	48
XPies (9 Inch):				
Apple	1/8 pie	13	4	15
Butterscotch	1/8 pie	13	4	11
Cherry	1/8 pie	13	4	16
Custard	1/8 pie	13	3.5	14
Lemon Meringue	1/8 pie	11	3.5	13
Pecan	1/8 pie	24	6	10
Pumpkin	1/8 pie	13	3.5	11
XPumpkin Pie Mix, Canned	1 cup	0	4	24
XPopsicle	1 twin bar	0	1.5	?-
XPuddings:				
Chocolate, Made From Mix With Whole Milk:				
Instant	1/2 cup	5	2.5	22
Noninstant	1/2 cup	5	2.5	8
Vanilla, Made From Mix With Whole Milk:				
Instant	1/2 cup	4	2.5	18
Noninstant	1/2 cup	4	2.5	9
XSherbet, Orange	1/2 cup	2	2	2
XSugar:				
Brown, Packed	1/4 cup	0	3	1
White, Granulated	1/4 cup	0	2.5	0
White, Granulated	1 tablespoon	0	0.5	0
XSweet Roll:				
Danish Pastry, Commercial, Plain	1 (4" x 1")	15	3.5	10
Cinnamon Rasin From Refrigerator Dough	2 pastries	14	5.5	19
XSyrup:				
Corn, Light & Dark	1 tablespoon	0	1	1
Can Maple Blend	1 tablespoon	0	0.5	0

MISCELLANEOUS

FOOD	SERVING SIZE	FAT GRAMS	CALORIE POINTS	SODIUM POINTS
Baking Powder:				
Regular	1 teaspoon	0	0	13
Low Sodium	1 teaspoon	0	0	0

FOOD	SERVING SIZE	FAT GRAMS	CALORIE POINTS	SODIUM POINTS
Baking Soda	1 teaspoon	0	0	36
Beverages:				
Alcoholic:				
Beer, Regular	12 ounces	0	2	1
Beer, Light	12 ounces	0	1.5	0
Bloody Mary Cocktail	5 ounces	0	1.5	14
X Daiquiri	2 ounces	0	1.5	0
Martini, No Olives	2.5 ounces	0	2	0
X Pina Colada	4.5 ounces	0	3.5	0
Gin, Rum, Vodka,				
Whiskey	1.5 ounces	0	1.5	0
X Coffee Liqueur	1.5 ounces	0	2.5	0
X Creme De Menthe	1.5 ounces	0	2.5	0
X Wine:				
Table, All	3.5 ounces	0	1	0
Dessert, All	2 ounces	0	1.5	0
Cooler	12 ounces	0	3	0
Carbonated:				
Club Soda	12 ounces	0	0	3
X Cream Soda	12 ounces	0	2.5	2
X Cola Type	12 ounces	0	2	1
Diet Soda, Cola,				
With Aspartame	12 ounces	0	0	1
X Ginger Ale	12 ounces	0	1.5	1
X Grape	12 ounces	0	2	2
X Lemon-Lime	12 ounces	0	2	2
Mineral Water	12 ounces	0	0	0
X Orange	12 ounces	0	2.5	2
X Pepper-Type	12 ounces	0	2	2
X Root Beer	12 ounces	0	2	2
X Tonic Or Quinine	12 ounces	0	1.5	1
X Cocoa Mix, With Added				
Nutrients, Powder	1 packet	1	1.5	9
X Instant Breakfast, Vanilla	1 envelope	0	2	6
X Orange Flavor Drink				
Powder	3 rounded tsp.	0	1.5	0
Coffee:				
Brewed	Any amount	0	0	0
Flavors From Instant:				
Cappucino	2 rounded tsp.	2	1	4
French	2 rounded tsp.	3	1	?−
Plain Powder	Any amount	0	0	0
Tea:				
Brewed	Any amount	0	0	0
Plain Powder	Any amount	0	0	0
X Lemon Powder With				
Sugar	3 rounded tsp.	0	0	?−
X Catsup, Tomato	2 tablespoons	0	0.5	15
Chocolate, Baking Or Bitter	1 ounce	15	2	0

FOOD	SERVING SIZE	FAT GRAMS	CALORIE POINTS	SODIUM POINTS
Cocoa, Dry Powder, Not Dutch Process	2 tablespoons	1	0	0
Cream Of Tartar	1 teaspoon	0	0	9
Gelatin, Unflavored, Dry	1 envelope	0	0.5	0
Gravies:				
Dehydrated, Au Jus	1 packet	3	1	104
Horseradish	1 teaspoon	0	0	0
XInstant Breakfast, Vanilla	1 envelope	0	2	6
Mustard, Prepared, Yellow	1 teaspoon	0	0	3
Nuts And Seeds:				
Almond Kernels, Whole, Dried, Unblanched, Unsalted	1 ounce (24)	15	2.5	0
Brazilnut Kernels, Large, Dried, Unsalted	1 ounce (6)	19	2.5	0
Cashew Nut Kernels, Medium, Oil Roasted, Salted	1 ounce (18)	14	2	8
X Coconut Meat, Sweetened, Flaked, Packaged	1/4 cup	6	1	2
Mixed Nuts With Peanuts:				
Dry Roasted, Salted	1/4 cup	18	3	10
Oil Roasted, Salted	1/4 cup	20	3	10
Peanuts, Oil Roasted:				
Salted	1/4 cup	20	3	7
Unsalted	1/4 cup	20	3	0
Peanuts, Dry Roasted, Salted	1/4 cup	18	3	13
Pecan Halves, Large, Dried, Unsalted	1 ounce (31)	19	2	0
Sesame Seeds, Unsalted	2 tablespoons	9	1.5	0
Sunflower Seeds, Unsalted	1/4 cup	18	3	0
Walnuts, Dried, Unsalted, Black Or English	1/4 cup	19	2.5	0
Olives, Pitted:				
Green	10 (.75" x 1")	5	0.5	40
Ripe	10 (.75" x 1")	5	0.5	17
Pickles:				
Dill	1 large (3.75" long)	0	0	36
Dill	2 slices	0	0	7
X Sweet Gherkin	1 large (3" long)	0	0.5	14
XSweet Relish	1 tablespoon	0	0.5	5
Salt, Lite	1/4 teaspoon	0	0	12
Salt, Table	1 teaspoon	0	0	100
Salt Substitute	1/4 teaspoon	0	0	0

FOOD	SERVING SIZE	FAT GRAMS	CALORIE POINTS	SODIUM POINTS
Sauces:				
Barbecue	1/4 cup	0	0.5	22
Salsa, Pace	2 teaspoons	0	0	4
Soy	1 tablespoon	0	0	45
Teriyaki	1 tablespoon	0	0	30
Worcestershire	1 tablespoon	0	0	10
Snack Foods:				
Apple Chips	1 ounce	5	1.5	1
Cheese Balls/Curls	1 ounce	11	2	12
Cheez Doodles	1 ounce	9	2	16
Chex Party Mix, Ralston	2/3 cup	5	1.5	14
Corn Chips	1 ounce	9	2	9
Dips, Home Recipes, Lower Fat Ingredients:				
Cocktail Crab	1/4 cup	7	1.5	7
Spinach	1/4 cup	1	0.5	1
Salmon Yogurt	1/4 cup	4	2	13
Dips, Commercial, Kraft:				
Avocado	1/4 cup	8	1.5	18
Clam	1/4 cup	8	1.5	21
Blue Cheese	1/4 cup	8	1	17
Nacho Cheese	1/4 cup	8	1.5	17
Jalapeno Bean	1/4 cup	8	1.5	14
Popcorn, Popped, Large Kernel, Commercial:				
With Oil & Salt	3 cups	6	1.5	23
Plain	3 cups	1	1	0
Popcorn, Popped, Microwavable:				
Pop Secret Light, Betty Crocker	3 cups	1	0.5	3
Light, Orville Redenbacher	3 cups	3	1	5
Pork Rinds	1 ounce	9	2	23
Potato:				
Chips	1 ounce	10	2	6
Pringles	1 ounce	13	2.5	9
Ruffles Light	1 ounce	6	2	6
Sticks	1 ounce	10	2	3
Pretzels	1 ounce	1	1.5	20
Soups:				
Commercial, Canned:				
Cream Type Condensed:				
Cheese	1 can	25	5	101
Chicken	1 can	18	4	104
Mushroom	1 can	23	4	107
Tomato	1 can	5	3	92
Prepared With Milk:				
Mushroom	1 cup	14	2.5	47
Pea, Green	1 cup	7	3	46
Potato	1 cup	6	2	50

FOOD	SERVING SIZE	FAT GRAMS	CALORIE POINTS	SODIUM POINTS
Soups, Commercial, Canned:				
Made With Milk:				
Tomato	1 cup	6	2	41
Prepared With Water:				
Chicken Noodle	1 cup	2	1	44
Vegetable/Beef	1 cup	2	1	42
Dehydrated Form:				
Broth Or Bouillon:				
Beef	1 cube	0	0	38
Beef	1 packet	1	0	44
Chicken	1 cube	0	0	50
Onion Mix	1 packet	2	1.5	152
Tartar Sauce	1 tablespoon	9	1	4
Tofu, Raw, Firm	1/2 cup	11	2.5	0
Vinegar, Cider	Any amount	0	0	0

COMBINATION AND CONVENIENCE FOODS

FOOD	SERVING SIZE	FAT GRAMS	CALORIE POINTS	SODIUM POINTS
Beef Vegetable Stew, Homemade, No Salt	1 cup	11	3	4
Bucket Dinners, Lunch				
Bucket:				
Chicken & Vegetables	1 (8.5 oz.)	8	3	42
Chili Mac	1 (8.5 oz.)	15	3.5	60
Chicken A La King, Homemade	1 cup	34	6.5	33
Chicken & Noodles, Homemade	1 cup	19	5	26
Chicken Tonight Sauces, Ragu:				
Creamy With Mushrooms	1 serving (1/6 jar)	10	1.5	27
Herb With Wine	1 serving (1/6 jar)	4	1.5	27
Salsa	1 serving (1/6 jar)	0	0.5	30
Chili Con Carne With Beans:				
Canned	1 cup	14	4	58
Homemade, Lean beef	1 cup	4	2.5	33
Chop Suey, Beef, Homemade	1 cup	17	4	46
Chow Mein, Chicken Homemade	1 cup	10	3	31
Corned Beef Hash, Armour	1/2 can (15 oz.)	27	5.5	39
Egg Rolls, Cantonese, Frozen, Van De Kamp	5.25 ounces	5	4	24
Enchiladas, Beef, Frozen, Van De Kamp	4 enchiladas	15	4.5	64
Frozen Dinners, Banquet:				
Beef, Chopped	1 dinner (11oz.)	30	6	52
Chicken, Fried	1 dinner (11oz.)	11	5	80
Helper Dinners:				
Chicken & Other Ingredients	1 serving (1/5 pkg.)	28	7	51

FOOD	SERVING SIZE	FAT GRAMS	CALORIE POINTS	SODIUM POINTS
Helper Dinners:				
Hamburger & Added Ingredients	1 serving (1/5 pkg.)	15	4.5	42
Tuna & Added Ingredients	1 serving (1/5 pkg.)	11	4	43
La Choy, Chinese, Canned Items:				
Pepper Steak, Dinner Classic, Oriental Vegetables, Sauce Mix, Added Ground Beef	3/4 cup prepared	9	2.5	47
Crispy Wide Noodles	1/2 cup	8	2	13
Fried Rice	3/4 cup	1	2.5	39
Lasagna, With Meat, Frozen, Van De Kamp	11 ounces	25	6	42
Macaroni & Cheese:				
Frozen	9 ounce meal	16	4.5	41
Boxed, Prepared	3/4 cup	13	3.5	28
Microwave Meals:				
Chef Boyardee:				
Cheese Ravioli	1 (7.5 oz.)	3	2.5	?-
Spaghetti/Meat Balls	1 (7.5 oz.)	10	3	?-
Chef Boyardee, Mini:				
Ravioli	1 can (15 oz.)	10	5.5	?-
Mini Bites	1 can (15 oz.)	24	7	?-
Hormel Micro Cup:				
Spaghetti/Meat Balls	1 (7.5 oz.)	7	2.5	?-
Chili Mac	1 (7.5 oz.)	10	2.5	?-
Kraft Microwavable Entrees:				
Spaghetti & Meat Sauce	1 meal	13	4.5	54
Sweet & Sour Chicken	1 meal	2	3	38
Top Shelf, Hormel:				
Vegetable Lasagna	1 meal	9	4	42
Spaghetti & Meat Sauce	1 meal	6	3.5	43
Pizza Crust Mix & Sauce:				
Appian Way	1/4 package (12.5 oz. pkg.)	3	2.5	25
Chef Boyardee	1/4 package (13.5 oz. pkg.)	3	2.5	28
Pizza, Frozen With Cheese, Totino's Classic	1/4 pizza	15	4.5	35
Pizza Quick Sauce, Ragu:				
Mushroom Or Traditional	3 tablespoons	2	0.5	14
Pepperoni	3 tablespoons	3	0.5	14
Pot Pie, Frozen, Banquet:				
Beef	8 ounces	24	6	56
Chicken	8 ounces	24	6	42
Ravioli, Beef, In Sauce, Canned, FrancoAmerican	7.5 ounces	5	3	47

FOOD	SERVING SIZE	FAT GRAMS	CALORIE POINTS	SODIUM POINTS
Rice-A-Roni, Chicken Flavor	1/6 package (6.9 oz pkg.)	0	1.5	21
Rice & Sauce, Lipton:				
Chicken Flavor	1/4 package	1	1.5	22
Herb & Butter	1/4 package	2	2	19
Rice & Beans, Cajun	1/4 package	0	1.5	26
Spaghetti, Canned:				
SpaghettiOs, Franco-American	1 can (15 ounces)	4	5	70
Cheese Or Meat, Heinz	1 can (15.5 ounces)	8	4.5	90
Tuna Noodle Casserole, Homemade	1.5 cups	7	4	?–

FREE FOODS

Unsalted Bouillon Cubes or Broth Or Regular Bouillon Or Broth, If Sodium Is Not A Concern
Seltzer Water (No Salt Or Sodium)
Coffee, Black, Unsweetened
Coffee, Decaffeinated, Black, Unsweetened
"Diet" Carbonated Beverages
Low Sodium Dill Pickles
Most Flavoring Essences
Horseradish
Herbs
Low Sodium Mustard Or Regular Mustard, If Sodium Is Not A Concern
Pimiento, Unsalted Canned
Spices
Tabasco Sauce
Tea, Unsweetened
Vinegar

NOTE: The primary source of food value information for the fat grams, calorie and sodium points on the preceding pages was the U.S. Department of Agriculture Handbook #8, COMPOSITION OF FOODS, Nos. 1, 4, 5, 6, 7, 8, 9, 10, 11, 12, 13, 14, 15, 16, 17, 19, 20 and the 1989 and 1990 Supplements. Other sources were Pennington, J.A.T. and Church, H.N., Bowes & Church's FOOD VALUES OF PORTIONS COMMONLY USED, Fifteenth Edition, 1989, Philadelphia: J.B. Lippincott Company, and information from food manufacturing companies.

FOOD	SERVING SIZE	FAT GRAMS	CALORIE POINTS	SODIUM POINTS
FAST FOODS				
ARBY'S®[1]				
Breakfast Items:				
Toastix	1 serving	25	5.5	19
X Maple Syrup	1 serving	0	1.5	2
X Cinnamon Nut Danish	1	11	5	5
Biscuit:				
Plain	1	15	4	32
Bacon	1	18	4.5	39
Sausage	1	32	6	43
Ham	1	17	4.5	51
Croissant:				
Plain	1	16	3.5	13
Bacon/Egg	1	30	6	31
Ham/Cheese	1	21	4.5	41
Mushroom/Cheese	1	38	6.5	41
Sausage/Egg	1	39	7	27
Platters:				
Ham	1	26	7	51
Sausage	1	41	8.5	37
Egg	1	24	6	26
Bacon	1	33	8	38
X Blueberry Muffin	1	7	3	9
Roast Beef Sandwiches:				
Regular	1	18	5	41
Beef 'N Cheddar	1	27	7	51
Junior	1	11	3	23
Giant	1	26	7.5	62
Super	1	28	7.5	51
Philly Beef 'N Swiss	1	25	6.5	50
Roast Beef Sandwiches:				
Bac 'N Cheddar Deluxe	1	32	7	48
French Dip	1	15	5	44
French Dip 'N Swiss	1	19	6	63
Arby Q	1	15	5.5	55
Chicken Sandwiches:				
Breast Fillet	1	23	6	42
Roast Club	1	27	7	50
Cordon Bleu	1	27	7	64
Grilled Deluxe	1	20	6	39
Grilled Barbecue	1	13	5	44
Other Sandwiches:				
Fish Fillet	1	27	7	38
Ham 'N Cheese	1	14	5	61
Arby's Sub Shop:				
Italian Sub	1	39	9	90
Roast Beef Sub	1	32	8.5	80
Tuna Sub	1	37	9	58
Turkey Sub	1	19	6.5	88

Arby's

FOOD	SERVING SIZE	FAT GRAMS	CALORIE POINTS	SODIUM POINTS
Light Sandwiches:				
Roast Beef Deluxe	1	10	4	36
Roast Turkey Deluxe	1	6	3.5	55
Roast Chicken Deluxe	1	7	3.5	34
Potatoes:				
French Fries	1 serving	13	3.5	5
Potato Cakes	1 serving	12	3	17
Curly Fries	1 serving	18	4.5	7
Cheddar Fries	1 serving	22	5.5	19
Baked:				
Plain	1	2	3	3
With Butter/Margarine & Sour Cream	1	25	6.5	9
Broccoli & Cheese	1	18	5.5	16
Deluxe	1	36	8.5	26
Mushroom 'N Cheese	1	27	7	40
Salads:				
Garden	1	5	1.5	6
Roast Chicken	1	7	3	22
Chef	1	10	3	35
Side	1	0	0.5	1
Salad Dressings:				
X Honey French	1 serving	27	4.5	21
Light Italian	1 serving	1	0.5	48
Thousand Island	1 serving	29	4	21
Blue Cheese	1 serving	31	4	21
Buttermilk Ranch	1 serving	39	4.5	20
Croutons	1 tablespoon	2	1	7
Soups:				
Boston Clam Chowder	1 serving	10	2.5	45
Cream Of Broccoli	1 serving	7	2	46
Lumberjack Mixed Vegetable	1 serving	4	1	47
Old Fashioned Chicken Noodle	1 serving	2	1.5	40
Potato With Bacon	1 serving	9	2.5	46
Wisconsin Cheese	1 serving	18	4	47
XDesserts:				
Apple Turnover	1	18	4	8
Cherry Turnover	1	18	4	9
Blueberry Turnover	1	19	4.5	10
Cheese Cake	1	23	4	10
Chocolate Chip Cookie	1	4	2	4
Chocalate Shake	1	12	6	15
Vanilla Shake	1	12	4.5	12
Jamocha Shake	1	11	5	11
Peanut Butter Cup Polar Swirl	1	24	7	17
Oreo Polar Swirl	1	20	6.5	23
Snickers Polar Swirl	1	19	7	15

FOOD	SERVING SIZE	FAT GRAMS	CALORIE POINTS	SODIUM POINTS
XDesserts:				
Heath Polar Swirl	1	22	7.5	15
Butterfinger Polar Swirl	1	18	6	14
Condiments:				
Arby's Sauce	1 serving	0	0	5
Horsey Sauce	1 serving	5	0.5	5
Ketchup	1 serving	0	0	6
Mustard	1 serving	1	0	7
Mayonnaise P.C.	1 serving	10	1	3
Au Jus	1 serving	0	0	33

BASKIN-ROBBINS®[1]

FOOD	SERVING SIZE	FAT GRAMS	CALORIE POINTS	SODIUM POINTS
XIce Cream:				
Chocolate Rasberry Truffle	1 scoop	17	4	5
Vanilla	1 scoop	14	3	5
Very Berry Strawberry	1 scoop	10	3	4
World Class Chocolate	1 scoop	14	4	6
XSherbet And Ices:				
Daiquiri Ice	1 scoop	0	2	1
Rainbow Sherbet	1 scoop	2	2	4
XNovelties—Sundae Bars:				
Light/Chocolate With Caramel Ribbon	1	5	2	3
Pralines 'N Cream	1	13	4	6
XVanilla Chilly Burgers	1	11	3	6
XTiny Toon Adventures Ice Cream Bar:				
Vanilla	1	14	3	2
Mint Chocolate Chip	1	15	3	2
X Cones:				
Sugar	1	1	1	2
Waffle	1	2	2	0
XFat Free With Simplesse, Chocolate Vanilla Twist Or				
Just Peachy	1/2 cup	0	1.5	3
Sugar Free With Nutrasweet:				
Jamoca Swiss Almond	1/2 cup	2	1	4
Strawberry	1/2 cup	1	1	3
XLight:				
Praline Dream	1/2 cup	6	2	4
Strawberry Royal	1/2 cup	1	1.5	5
XFrozen Yogurt:				
Low-Fat Strawberry	1/2 cup	1	1.5	2
Non-Fat Strawberry	1/2 cup	0	1.5	2
XStrawberry Soft-Serve				
Sorbet	1/2 cup	0	1.5	1

FOOD	SERVING SIZE	FAT GRAMS	CALORIE POINTS	SODIUM POINTS
BURGER KING®1				
Burgers:				
Whopper Sandwich	1	36	8.5	38
Whopper Sandwich With Cheese	1	44	9.5	51
Double Whopper Sandwich	1	53	11	41
Double Whopper, Cheese	1	61	12	54
Cheeseburger	1	15	4.5	29
Cheeseburger Deluxe	1	23	5.5	28
Hamburger	1	11	3.5	22
Hamburger Deluxe	1	19	4.5	22
Bacon Double Cheeseburger	1	30	7	35
Burgers:				
Bacon Double Cheeseburger Deluxe	1	38	8	38
Double Cheeseburger	1	27	6.5	37
Burger Buddies (Pair)	1 serving	17	4.5	31
Sandwiches And Side Orders:				
BK Broiler Chicken Sandwich	1	8	3.5	32
Chicken Sandwich	1	40	9	62
Ocean Catch Fish Filet Sandwich	1	33	6.5	32
Chicken Tenders	1	13	3	24
Chef Salad, No Dressing	1	9	2.5	25
Chunky Chicken Salad	1	4	2	19
Garden Salad	1	5	1.5	5
Side Salad	1	0	0.5	1
French Fries, Medium Salted	1 serving	20	5	10
Onion Rings	1 serving	19	4.5	27
X Apple Pie	1 serving	14	4	18
X Cherry Pie	1 serving	13	5	9
X Lemon Pie	1 serving	8	4	5
X Snickers Ice Cream Bar	1	14	3	3
X Drinks:				
Vanilla Shake	1	10	4.5	9
Chocolate Shake	1	10	4.5	9
Chocolate Shake (Syrup Added)	1	11	5.5	11
Strawberry Shake (Syrup Added)	1	10	5.5	10
Coca-Cola, Medium	22 ounces	0	3.5	?-
Sprite, Medium	22 ounces	0	3.5	?-

FOOD	SERVING SIZE	FAT GRAMS	CALORIE POINTS	SODIUM POINTS
Breakfast:				
Croissan'wich:				
With Bacon, Egg & Cheese	1	23	5	34
With Sausage, Egg & Cheese	1	40	7	43
With Ham, Egg & Cheese	1	22	4.5	60
Breakfast Buddy With Sausage, Egg & Cheese	1	16	3.5	21
French Toast Sticks	1 serving	32	7.5	23
Hash Browns	1 serving	12	3	14
X Mini Muffins, Blueberry	1	14	4	11
Condiments & Toppings:				
Mayonnaise	1 serving	21	2.5	6
Tartar Sauce	1 serving	14	2	9
BK Broiler Sauce	1 serving	4	0.5	3
Bull's Eye Barbecue Sauce	1 serving	0	0.5	2
Bacon Bits	1 teaspoon	1	0.5	?–
Croutons	1/4 ounce	1	0.5	4
Newman's Own Salad Dressings:				
Thousand Island	1 serving	26	4	18
French	1 serving	22	4	17
Ranch	1 serving	37	4.5	14
Bleu Cheese	1 serving	32	4	22
Olive Oil/Vinegar	1 serving	33	4	9
Reduced Calorie Light Italian	1 serving	18	2.5	33
Dipping Sauces:				
A.M. Express Dip	1 serving	0	1	1
X Honey Express Dip	1 serving	0	1	1
Ranch Dipping Sauce	1 serving	18	2.5	9
Barbecue Dipping Sauce	1 serving	0	0.5	17
X Sweet & Sour Dipping Sauce	1 serving	0	0.5	2

CAPTAIN D'S®[1]

Broiled & Baked Dinners (Includes rice, green beans, bread stick, salad and low calorie Italian Dressing):

FOOD	SERVING SIZE	FAT GRAMS	CALORIE POINTS	SODIUM POINTS
Orange Roughy Dinner	1	19	7	94
Shrimp Dinner	1	10	6	95
Chicken Dinner	1	8	5.5	114
Baked Fish Dinner	1	9	7	94
Other Broiled Dinners (Availability Varies):				
Halibut Dinner	1	10	6	92
Swordfish Dinner	1	13	6.5	95
Trout Dinner	1	11	6	90

FOOD	SERVING SIZE	FAT GRAMS	CALORIE POINTS	SODIUM POINTS
Other Broiled Dinners:				
Mixed Grill (Salmon, Tuna, Swordfish) Dinner	1	13	7	93
Tuna Dinner	1	14	7	91
Flounder Dinner	1	9	6.5	95
Grouper Dinner	1	9	6.5	93
Ocean Perch Dinner	1	10	6.5	95
Side Items:				
Cracklins	1 ounce	17	3	32
French Fried Potatoes	1 serving	10	4	7
Cole Slaw	1 serving	12	2	11
Cole Slaw	1 pint	47	8.5	20
Green Beans, Seasoned	1 serving	2	0.5	33
White Beans	1 serving	1	1.5	4
Rice	1 serving	0	1.5	0
Fried Okra	1 serving	16	4	19
Hushpuppy	1	4	1.5	20
Hushpuppies	6	25	10	121
Breadstick	1	1	1	9
Breadsticks	6	7	7.5	55
Dinner Salad, No Dressing	1 serving	1	0.5	3
Dressings:				
French	1 packet	11	1.5	8
Blue Cheese	1 packet	12	1.5	4
Ranch	1 packet	10	1	10
Low Calorie Italian	1 packet	0	0	25
Crackers	4	1	0.5	6
Slice of Cheese	1	5	0.5	9
Cocktail Sauce	1 side portion	0	0.5	11
Cocktail Sauce	1 bulk portion	0	2	44
Tartar Sauce	1 side portion	7	1	7
Tartar Sauce	1 bulk portion	27	4	28
X Sweet & Sour Sauce	1 side portion	0	0.5	0
X Sweet & Sour Sauce	1 bulk portion	0	3	1
Nondairy Creamer	2 creamers	2	0.5	16
XDesserts:				
Pecan Pie	1 piece	20	6	16
Chocolate Cake	1 piece	10	4	11
Carrot Cake	1 piece	23	6	18
Cheesecake	1 piece	31	5.5	21
Lemon Pie	1 piece	10	4.5	6
DAIRY QUEEN®[1]				
XBlizzards:				
Strawberry, Small	1 serving	12	7	7
Strawberry, Regular	1 serving	16	10	10
Heath, Small	1 serving	23	7.5	12
Heath, Regular	1 serving	36	11	18

FOOD	SERVING SIZE	FAT GRAMS	CALORIE POINTS	SODIUM POINTS
XBreezes:				
Strawberry, Small	1 serving	0	5.5	5
Strawberry, Regular	1 serving	1	8	7
Heath, Small	1 serving	12	6	10
Heath, Regular	1 serving	21	9	16
XCones:				
Vanilla, Small	1 cone	4	2	3
Vanilla, Regular	1 cone	7	3	4
Vanilla, Large	1 cone	10	4.5	6
Chocolate, Regular	1 cone	7	3	5
Chocolate, Large	1 cone	11	4.5	7
Chocolate, Regular, Dipped	1 cone	16	4.5	4
Yogurt, Regular	1 cone	0	2.5	3
Yogurt, Large	1 cone	0	3.5	5
XCups And Scoops:				
QC Vanilla, Big	1 scoop	14	4	4
QC Chocolate, Big	1 scoop	14	4	4
Yogurt, Regular	1 cup	0	2.5	3
Yogurt, Large	1 cup	0	3	4
XMiscellaneous Desserts:				
Banana Split	1	11	7	11
Buster Bar	1	29	6	10
Dilly Bar	1	13	3	2
DQ Sandwich	1	4	2	6
DQ Frozen Cake Slice	1	18	5	9
Hot Fudge Brownie Delight	1	29	9.5	15
Nutty Double Fudge	1	22	8	7
Peanut Buster Parfait	1	32	9.5	18
XMr. Misty, Regular	1 serving	0	3.5	0
XShakes:				
Vanilla, Regular	1	14	7	10
Vanilla, Large	1	16	8	11
Chocolate, Regular	1	14	7.5	13
Vanilla Malt, Regular	1	14	8	10
XSundaes:				
Chocolate, Regular	1 serving	7	4	6
Strawberry Waffle Cone	1 serving	12	4.5	10
Strawberry Yogurt, Regular	1 serving	0	2.5	3
Sandwiches:				
Hamburger:				
Single	1	13	4	25
Single With Cheese	1	18	5	35
Double	1	25	6	27
Double With Cheese	1	34	7.5	47
DQ Homestyle, Ultimate	1	47	9.5	48

Dairy Queen

FOOD	SERVING SIZE	FAT GRAMS	CALORIE POINTS	SODIUM POINTS
Sandwiches:				
Hot Dog:				
Regular	1	16	4	30
With Cheese	1	21	4.5	40
With Chili	1	19	4.5	31
1/4# Super Dog	1	38	8	59
BBQ Beef	1	4	3	30
Grilled Chicken Fillet	1	8	4	35
Breaded Chicken Fillet	1	20	6	33
With Cheese	1	25	6.5	43
Fish Fillet	1	16	5	27
With Cheese	1	21	5.5	37
Salads:				
Side, No Dressing	1 serving	0	0.5	1
Garden, No Dressing	1 serving	13	2.5	10
Dressings:				
Thousand Island	1 serving	21	3	25
Reduced Calorie French	1 serving	5	1	20
French Fries:				
Small	1 serving	10	3	5
Regular	1 serving	14	4	7
Large	1 serving	18	5.5	9
Onion Rings, Regular	1 serving	12	3	6

GODFATHER'S PIZZA®[1]

FOOD	SERVING SIZE	FAT GRAMS	CALORIE POINTS	SODIUM POINTS
Original Crust:				
Cheese Pizza:				
Mini	1/4 pizza	4	2	7
Small	1/6 pizza	7	3	13
Medium	1/8 pizza	7	3.5	12
Large	1/10 pizza	8	3.5	14
Combo Pizza:				
Mini	1/4 pizza	5	2	12
Small	1/6 pizza	11	4	25
Medium	1/8 pizza	12	4.5	25
Large	1/10 pizza	12	4.5	27
Golden Crust:				
Cheese Pizza:				
Small	1/6 pizza	8	3	11
Medium	1/8 pizza	9	3	12
Large	1/10 pizza	11	3.5	14
Combo Pizza:				
Small	1/6 pizza	12	3.5	24
Medium	1/8 pizza	13	4	23
Large	1/10 pizza	15	4.5	26

FOOD	SERVING SIZE	FAT GRAMS	CALORIE POINTS	SODIUM POINTS
HARDEES®¹				
Breakfast Menu:				
Biscuit:				
Rise 'N Shine	1	18	4.5	32
X Cinnamon 'N Raisin	1	17	4.5	22
Sausage	1	28	6	48
Sausage & Egg	1	31	6.5	50
Bacon	1	21	5	41
Bacon & Egg	1	24	5.5	43
Bacon, Egg & Cheese	1	28	6	53
Ham	1	16	4.5	43
Ham & Egg	1	19	5	46
Ham, Egg & Cheese	1	23	5.5	55
Country Ham	1	18	4.5	67
Country Ham & Egg	1	22	5.5	70
Canadian Rise 'N Shine	1	27	6.5	67
Steak	1	29	7	57
Steak & Egg	1	32	7.5	60
Chicken	1	22	6	58
'N Gravy	1	24	6	54
Big Country Breakfast:				
Sausage	1	57	11	86
Bacon	1	40	9	67
Ham	1	33	8.5	77
Country Ham	1	38	9	125
Hash Rounds	1 serving	14	3	24
Pancakes & Accompaniments:				
Three	1 serving	2	4	39
Three With Sausage Patty	1 serving	16	6	56
Three With 2 Bacon Strips	1 serving	9	4.5	48
X Syrup	1 serving	0	1.5	1
Margarine/Butter Blend	1 teaspoon	4	0.5	2
Sandwiches:				
Hamburgers:				
Plain	1	10	3.5	21
Cheeseburger	1	14	4.5	31
Quarter-Pound With Cheese	1	29	7	46
Big Deluxe	1	30	7	33
Bacon & Cheese	1	39	8	45
Mushroom 'N Swiss	1	27	6.5	41
Big Twin	1	25	6	25
Roast Beef, Regular	1	9	3.5	32
Big Roast Beef	1	11	4	38
Hot Ham 'N Cheese	1	12	4.5	62
Turkey Club	1	16	5.5	56

FOOD	SERVING SIZE	FAT GRAMS	CALORIE POINTS	SODIUM POINTS
Sandwich:				
Fisherman's Fillet	1	24	7	45
Chicken Fillet	1	13	5	46
Grilled Chicken	1	9	4	39
All Beef Hotdog	1	17	4	31
Chicken Stix (6)	1 serving	9	3	30
Chicken Stix (9)	1 serving	14	4	44
French Fries:				
Regular	1 serving	11	3	4
Large	1 serving	17	5	6
Big Fry	1 serving	23	7	8
Crispy Curls	1 serving	16	4	37
Salads:				
Side (No Dressing)	1	0	0.5	1
Garden	1	14	3	12
Chef	1	15	3	40
Chicken 'N Pasta	1	3	3	17
XShakes And Desserts:				
Shakes:				
Vanilla	1	9	5.5	14
Chocolate	1	8	6	15
Strawberry	1	8	6	13
Cool Twist Cones:				
Vanilla	1	6	2.5	4
Chocolate	1	6	2.5	3
Vanilla/Chocolate	1	6	2.5	3
Cool Twist Sundaes:				
Hot Fudge	1	12	4.5	12
Caramel	1	10	4.5	13
Strawberry	1	8	3.5	5
AppleTurnover	1	12	3.5	11
Big Cookie	1	13	3.5	10

KFC®1 (Kentucky Fried Chicken)

FOOD	SERVING SIZE	FAT GRAMS	CALORIE POINTS	SODIUM POINTS
Original Recipe Chicken:				
Wing	1 piece	11	2.5	17
Side Breast	1 piece	15	3.5	26
Center Breast	1 piece	14	3.5	26
Drumstick	1 piece	9	2	12
Thigh	1 piece	21	4	26
Extra Tasty Crispy Chicken:				
Wing	1 piece	17	3	14
Side Breast	1 piece	27	5	28
Center Breast	1 piece	21	4.5	28
Drumstick	1 piece	14	3	13
Thigh	1 piece	31	5.5	25
Hot & Spicy Chicken:				
Wing	1 piece	18	3.5	20
Side Breast	1 piece	27	5.5	40

FOOD	SERVING SIZE	FAT GRAMS	CALORIE POINTS	SODIUM POINTS
Hot And Spicy Chicken:				
Center Breast	1 piece	25	5	39
Drumstick	1 piece	14	3	18
Thigh	1 piece	30	5.5	33
Lite 'N Crispy Chicken:				
Side Or Center Breast	1 piece	12	3	18
Drumstick	1 piece	7	1.5	9
Thigh	1 piece	17	3.5	17
Chicken Littles	1	10	2.5	14
Buttermilk Biscuits	1	12	3	28
Mashed Potatoes & Gravy	1 serving	2	1	15
French Fries	1 serving	12	3.5	6
Crispy Fries	1 serving	17	4	33
Corn-On-The-Cob	1 serving	2	1	0
Coleslaw	1 serving	6	1.5	8
Colonel's Chicken Sandwich	1	27	6.5	46
Hot Wings	1 serving (6)	33	6.5	53
Kentucky Nuggets:				
Kentucky Nuggets	1 serving (6)	18	4	38
Kentucky Nuggets Sauces:				
Barbecue	1 serving	1	0.5	20
X Sweet 'N Sour	1 serving	1	1	6
X Honey	1 serving	0	0.5	1
Mustard	1 serving	1	0.5	15

LONG JOHN SILVER'S®[1]

FOOD	SERVING SIZE	FAT GRAMS	CALORIE POINTS	SODIUM POINTS
Standard Entrees, Baked:				
Fish, Lemon Crumb, Rice, Green Beans, Slaw, Roll	3 piece dinner	12	7.5	64
Fish, Lemon Crumb, Light Portion, Rice, Small Salad, No Dressing	2 piece dinner	5	3.5	30
Chicken, Rice, Green Beans, Slaw, Roll	1 dinner	15	7.5	73
Ala Carte, Baked:				
Fish, Lemon Crumb	3 pieces	1	2	16
Chicken, Light Herb	1 serving	4	1.5	25
Sandwiches, Without Sauce:				
Batter-Dipped Fish	1 piece sandwich	15	4.5	34
Batter-Dipped Chicken	2 piece sandwich	16	5.5	47
Standard Entrees:				
Fish, Fries, Slaw, 2 Hushpuppies	2 piece dinner	48	12	78
Fish, Fries	2 piece dinner	37	8	64
Chicken Planks, Fries, 2 Hushpuppies, Slaw	3 piece dinner	44	12	87
Chicken Planks, Fries	2 piece dinner	26	6.5	56

KFC and Long John Silver's

FOOD	SERVING SIZE	FAT GRAMS	CALORIE POINTS	SODIUM POINTS
Standard Entrees:				
Clams, Fries, Slaw, 2 Hushpuppies	1 dinner	52	13	80
Shrimp, Fries, Slaw	10 piece dinner	47	11	71
Fish (1), Chicken (1), Fries	1 dinner	32	7.5	60
Fish (1), Chicken (2), Fries, Slaw, 2 Hushpuppies	1 dinner	49	12.5	91
Fish (1), Shrimp (8), Fries, Slaw, 2 Hushpuppies	1 dinner	65	15	106
Fish (2), Shrimp (5), Chicken (1), Fries, Slaw, 2 Hushpuppies	1 dinner	65	15.5	113
Fish (2), Shrimp (4), Clams (6 Oz.), Fries, Slaw, 2 Hushpuppies	1 dinner	70	16.5	114
Salads, No Dressing Or Crackers:				
Ocean Chef	1 salad	1	1.5	32
Seafood	1 salad	31	5	43
Small	1 salad	0	0	0
Standard Entrees, Kid's Meals:				
Fish (1), Fries, 1 Hushpuppy	1 dinner	28	7	44
Fish (1), Chicken (1), Fries, 1 Hushpuppy	1 dinner	34	8.5	61
Chicken Planks (2), Fries, 1 Hushpuppy	1 dinner	29	7.5	57
A-La-Carte Items:				
Batter-Dipped Fish	1 piece	11	2.5	21
Chicken Planks	1 piece	6	1.5	17
Batter-Dipped Shrimp	1 piece	2	0.5	3
Seafood Chowder With Cod	1 serving	6	2	26
Seafood Gumbo With Cod	1 serving	8	1.5	32
Fries	1 serving	15	3.5	22
Hushpuppy	1 piece	2	1	1
Corn Cobbette	1 piece	8	2	0
Green Beans	1 serving	0	0.5	14
Rice	1 serving	3	2	15
Cole Slaw	1 serving	6	2	11
Small Salad	1 serving	0	0.5	0
Roll	1	0	1.5	7
X Desserts:				
Lemon Pie	1 piece	9	4.5	6
Cherry Pie	1 piece	13	5	9

FOOD	SERVING SIZE	FAT GRAMS	CALORIE POINTS	SODIUM POINTS
X Desserts:				
Apple Pie	1 piece	13	4.5	18
Walnut Brownie	1 piece	22	6	7
Cookie:				
Oatmeal Raisin	1 cookie	10	2	7
Chocolate Chip	1 cookie	9	3	7
Condiments:				
Catsup	1 portion	0	0	6
Seafood Sauce	1 portion	0	0	8
Tartar Sauce	1 portion	5	0.5	2
X Honey Mustard Sauce	1 portion	0	0.5	3
Malt Vinegar	1 portion	0	0	1
X Sweet 'N Sour Sauce	1 portion	0	0.5	2
Ranch Dressing	1 portion	19	2.5	10
Creamy Italian Dressing	1 portion	3	0.5	12
Sea Salad Dressing	1 portion	15	2	7
Saltine Crackers	1 package	1	0.5	3

McDONALDS®[1]

FOOD	SERVING SIZE	FAT GRAMS	CALORIE POINTS	SODIUM POINTS
Breakfast:				
Egg McMuffin	1	11	4	31
Sausage McMuffin	1	20	4.5	33
Sausage McMuffin With Egg	1	25	6	40
English Muffin With Spread	1	4	2.5	12
Sausage Biscuit	1	28	5.5	45
Sausage Biscuit With Egg	1	33	7	53
Bacon, Egg & Cheese Biscuit	1	26	6	53
Biscuit With Biscuit Spread	1	13	3.5	32
Sausage	1 serving	15	2	13
Scrambled Eggs (2)	1 serving	10	2	13
Hash Brown Potatoes	1 serving	7	2	14
X Hotcakes, Margarine & Syrup	1 serving	12	6	30
Breakfast Burrito	1	17	4	25
X Fat-Free Apple Bran Muffin	1	0	2.5	9
X Apple Danish	1	17	5.5	16
X Iced Cheese Danish	1	21	5.5	18
X Cinnamon Raisin Danish	1	21	6	19
X Raspberry Danish	1	16	5.5	13
Sandwiches:				
Hamburger	1	9	3.5	21
Cheeseburger	1	13	4	32
Quarter Pounder	1	20	5.5	28

FOOD	SERVING SIZE	FAT GRAMS	CALORIE POINTS	SODIUM POINTS
Sandwiches:				
Quarterpounder				
With Cheese	1	28	7	48
McLean Deluxe	1	10	4.5	29
With Cheese	1	14	5	39
Big Mac	1	26	7	39
Filet-O-Fish	1	18	5	32
McChicken	1	20	5.5	36
Chicken Fajitas (1)	1	8	2.5	13
French Fries:				
Small	1 serving	12	3	5
Medium	1 serving	17	4.5	7
Large	1 serving	22	5.5	9
Chicken McNuggets/Sauces:				
Chicken McNuggets	1 serving (6)	15	3.5	25
Sauces:				
Hot Mustard	1 serving	4	1	11
Barbecue	1 serving	1	0.5	15
X Sweet 'N Sour	1 serving	0	1	8
X Honey	1 serving	0	0.5	0
Salads/Dressings/Accompaniments:				
Chef Salad	1	9	2.5	17
Chunky Chicken Salad	1	4	2	10
Garden Salad	1	2	0.5	3
Side Salad	1	1	0.5	2
Croutons	1 serving	2	0.5	6
Bacon Bits	1 serving	1	0	4
Bleu Cheese Dressing	1 packet	20	3.5	33
Lite Vinaigrette Dressing	1 packet	2	0.5	10
Ranch Dressing	1 packet	20	3	23
Red French Reduced				
Calorie Dressing	1 packet	8	2.5	20
1000 Island Dressing	1 packet	15	3	22
XDesserts/Milk Shakes:				
Vanilla Lowfat Frozen				
Yogurt Cone	1 cone (3 ounces)	1	1.5	3
Lowfat Frozen Yogurt Sundaes:				
Strawberry	1	1	3	4
Hot Fudge	1	3	3	7
Hot Caramel	1	3	3.5	8
Apple Pie	1 serving	15	3.5	10
Cookies:				
McDonaldland	1 serving	9	4	13
Chocolaty Chip	1 serving	15	4.5	12
Lowfat Milk Shakes:				
Chocolate	1	2	4.5	10
Strawberry	1	1	4.5	7
Vanilla	1	1	4	7

McDonald's

FOOD	SERVING SIZE	FAT GRAMS	CALORIE POINTS	SODIUM POINTS
PIZZA HUT®[1]				
Pan Pizza (Medium Size):				
Cheese	2 slices	18	6.5	41
Pepperoni	2 slices	22	7.5	49
Supreme	2 slices	30	8	59
Super Supreme	2 slices	26	7.5	63
Thin 'N Crispy Pizza (Medium Size):				
Cheese	2 slices	17	5.5	38
Pepperoni	2 slices	20	5.5	43
Supreme	2 slices	22	6	58
Super Supreme	2 slices	21	6.5	58
Hand Tossed (Medium Size):				
Cheese	2 slices	20	7	55
Pepperoni	2 slices	23	7	55
Supreme	2 slices	26	7.5	64
Super Supreme	2 slices	25	7.5	72
Personal Pan Pizza:				
Pepperoni	1 pizza	29	9	58
Supreme	1 pizza	28	8.5	57
SHONEY'S®[1]				
Breakfast Bar:				
Fruits & Vegetables (See Sections On Fruits & Vegetables)				
X Cold End:				
Sour Cream Brunch Cake	1 square	8	2	6
Apple Brunch Cake	1 square	8	2	7
Pineapple Brunch Cake	1 square	7	2	5
Banana Brunch Cake	1 square	7	2	5
Carrot Brunch Cake	1 square	7	2	7
Golden Pound Cake	1 slice	5	2	6
Marble Cake & Icing	1 slice	5	2	6
Jr. Honey Bun	1	5	2	3
Jr. Maple Bun	1	5	2	3
Jr. Chocolate Bun	1	5	2	3
Cinnamon Honey Bun	1	12	4.5	7
DoughNugget	1	10	2	8
Mini Cinnamon Donut	1	3	1	3
Powdered Sugar Donut	1	3	1	3
Shortcake	1	2	1	4
Bread Pudding	1 square	11	4	18
Hot End:				
X Syrup, Light	1 ladle	0	1	0
Pancakes	3	?-	1.5	12
Grits	1/4 cup	3	1	3
Country Gravy	1/4 cup	7	1	11
Cottage Fries	1/4 cup	2	1	5
Home Fries, Dices	1/2 cup	3	1.5	2
Hashbrowns	1/2 cup	3	1	2
Mushroom Topping	1 ounce	2	0.5	14

FOOD	SERVING SIZE	FAT GRAMS	CALORIE POINTS	SODIUM POINTS
Hot End:				
Omelette Topping	1 spoon	2	0.5	4
Cheese Sauce	1 ladle	2	0.5	7
Sausage Patty	1	13	2	?-
Sausage Link	1	9	1	13
Smoked Sausage	1	10	1.5	?-
Bacon	2 strips	6	1	8
Beef Stick	1	1	0.5	?-
Breakfast Ham	1 slice	1	0.5	11
Chicken Pieces	1 piece	2	0.5	?-
French Toast	1 piece	3	1	7
X Cereals:				
Captain Crunch Berry	1/2 cup	2	1	5
Raisin Bran	1/2 cup	1	1	7
Trix	1/2 cup	0	0.5	4
100 % Natural	1/2 cup	11	3.5	2
X Prepared Salads:				
Fruit Delight	1/2 cup	2	1.5	0
Fluff, Typical	1/2 cup	0	0.5	0
Breakfast Bar:				
X Cold End:				
Ambrosia	1/2 cup	7	2	15
Mixed Fruit	1/2 cup	0	1	0
Oriental	1/2 cup	5	2	3
Snow	1/2 cup	8	2	2
Waldorf	1/2 cup	10	2	6
Pistachio Pineapple	1/2 cup	5	2.5	3
Chocolate Pudding	1/2 cup	4	2	7
Glaced Fruit	1/2 cup	0	1.5	0
Apple Grape Surprise	1/2 cup	0	0.5	0
Toppings:				
X Fruit Topping	1 tablespoon	0	0.5	0
Whipped Topping	2 scoops	2	0.5	0
Cottage Cheese	3 tablespoons	1	0.5	9
Oleo, Whipped	1 tablespoon	8	1	4
X Apple Butter	1 tablespoon	0	0.5	0
X Grape Jelly	1 tablespoon	0	1	0
Kitchen Ordered Breakfasts:				
Pancakes (6" cake)	1	?-	1	23
Biscuit	1	8	2.5	16
Hashbrowns	3 ounces	3	1	2
Grits	3 ounces	3	1	3
Buttered Toast	2 slices	5	2	13
Bacon Strips	3	9	1.5	13
Egg, Fried	1	15	2	3
Sirloin Steak, Charbroiled	6 ounces	25	5	7
Home Fries	3 ounces	4	1.5	2
Sausage Patty	1	10	1.5	?-
Breakfast Ham	2 slices	2	1	23
Blueberry Muffin	2	7	3	?-

FOOD	SERVING SIZE	FAT GRAMS	CALORIE POINTS	SODIUM POINTS
Breakfast Side Items:				
X Jelly Packet	1	0	0.5	0
X Low-Cal Syrup	2 ounces	0	1.5	0
Country Gravy	3 ounces	10	1.5	16
X Honey Bun	1	14	3.5	1
Croissant	1	16	3.5	11
Salad Bar:				
Vegetables, No Dressing	As Desired	0	0	0
Green Olives	8	3	0.5	28
Black Olives	8	5	0.5	7
Fruits:				
Prunes	2 tablespoons	0	0.5	0
Apple Ring	2	0	0.5	0
Pineapple Bits	4 tablespoons	0	0.5	0
Grapefruit	1/4 cup	0	0.5	0
Breads & Garnishes:				
Bacon Bits	2 spoons	1	0.5	?–
Chow Mein Noodles	2 spoons	1	0.5	?–
Trail Mix	2 spoons	3	1	0
Sunflower Seeds	2 spoons	6	1	0
Croutons	2 spoons	1	0.5	3
Raisins	2 spoons	0	1	0
Granola	2 spoons	2	0.5	?–
Oil	1 teaspoon	5	0.5	0
Melba Toast	3 slices	0	0.5	2
Meat & Protein:				
Turkey Ham	2 tablespoons	1	0.5	11
Pepperoni	2 tablespoons	5	1	7
Diced Egg	2 tablespoons	2	0.5	1
Shredded Cheese	2 tablespoons	3	0.5	10
Cottage Cheese	2 tablespoons	0	0.5	6
Dressings:				
W.W. Italian	2 tablespoons	0	0	27
Biscayne Lo-Cal	2 tablespoons	1	1	15
Blue Cheese	2 tablespoons	13	1.5	5
Thousand Island	2 tablespoons	13	2	8
Ranch	2 tablespoons	10	1.5	?–
French	2 tablespoons	12	1.5	9
Rue French	2 tablespoons	10	1.5	16
Creamy Italian	2 tablespoons	15	2	20
Golden Italian	2 tablespoons	15	2	13
Honey Mustard	2 tablespoons	17	2	?–
Prepared Salads:				
X Mixed Fruit	1/4 cup	0	1	0
X Fruit Topping	1/4 cup	0	1	0
X Jello	1/4 cup	0	1	1
X Jello Fluff	1/4 cup	0	0.5	0
Macaroni	1/4 cup	14	1	17
Cucumber Lite	1/4 cup	0	0.5	15
Cole Slaw	1/4 cup	5	0.5	5

FOOD	SERVING SIZE	FAT GRAMS	CALORIE POINTS	SODIUM POINTS
Prepared Salads:				
Three Bean	1/4 cup	5	1	8
Pea	1/4 cup	6	1	4
Italian Vegetable	1/4 cup	0	0.5	5
Broccoli & Cauliflower	1/4 cup	9	1	21
Broccoli & Cauliflower, Ranch	1/4 cup	6	0.5	1
Rotelli Pasta	1/4 cup	4	0.5	4
Don's Pasta	1/4 cup	5	0.5	10
Spring	1/4 cup	3	0.5	7
Spaghetti	1/4 cup	5	1	?-
Ambrosia	1/4 cup	3	0.5	7
Summer	1/4 cup	12	0.5	10
Mixed Squash	1/4 cup	4	0.5	10
Broccoli, Cauliflower, & Carrot	1/4 cup	4	0.5	8
Oriental	1/4 cup	3	1	?-
Carrot Apple	1/4 cup	9	0.5	0
Fruit Delight	1/4 cup	2	1	0
Snow	1/4 cup	4	0.5	1
Beet Onion	1/4 cup	1	0.5	7
Kidney Bean	1/4 cup	2	0.5	7
Waldorf	1/4 cup	5	1	3
Pistachio Pineapple	1/4 cup	3	0.5	2
X Chocolate Pudding	1/4 cup	2	1	4
X Glaced Fruit	1/4 cup	0	1	0
Apple Grape Surprise	1/4 cup	0	0	0
Soups:				
Tomato Vegetable	6 ounces	0	0.5	14
Chicken Rice	6 ounces	1	1	5
Tomato Florentine	6 ounces	1	1	30
Bean	6 ounces	1	1	21
Cream of Chicken Vegetable	6 ounces	1	1	31
Chicken Noodle	6 ounces	1	1	6
Vegetable Beef	6 ounces	2	1	55
Chicken Gumbo	6 ounces	2	1	46
Onion	6 ounces	2	0.5	4
Cheddar Chowder	6 ounces	2	1	41
Beef Cabbage	6 ounces	3	1	22
Potato	6 ounces	3	1.5	15
Cream of Broccoli	6 ounces	5	1	18
Corn Chowder	6 ounces	5	2	22
Clam Chowder	6 ounces	5	1.5	?-
Cheese Florentine Ham	6 ounces	8	1.5	39
Cream Of Chicken	6 ounces	9	2	51
Broccoli & Cauliflower	6 ounces	9	1.5	24

FOOD	SERVING SIZE	FAT GRAMS	CALORIE POINTS	SODIUM POINTS
Menu Entrees:				
Charbroiled Steak & Chicken:				
Charbroiled Chicken	1 serving	7	3	26
Hawaiian Chicken	1 serving	7	3.5	26
Half 'O Pound	1 serving	34	6	12
Sirloin	6 ounces	25	5	7
Steak 'N Shrimp, Fried	1 serving	33	7	11
Steak 'N Shrimp, Charbroiled	1 serving	23	5	9
Ribeye	8 ounces	51	8	9
America's Favorites:				
Country Fried Steak	1 serving	27	6	51
Chicken Tenders	1 serving	20	5	10
Lasagna	1 serving	10	4	38
Spaghetti	1 serving	16	6.5	17
Liver 'N Onions	1 serving	23	5.5	14
Seafood:				
Shrimper's Feast	1 serving	22	5	9
Large Shrimper's Feast	1 serving	33	8	14
Bite-Size Shrimp	1 serving	25	5	55
Baked Fish	1 serving	1	2.5	71
Light Baked Fish	1 serving	1	2.5	71
Seafood Platter	1 serving	28	7.5	39
Charbroiled Shrimp	1 serving	3	2	7
Fish N' Shrimp	1 serving	26	6.5	28
Fish N' Chips, Fries	1 serving	35	8.5	38
Other Entrees:				
Light Beef Patty	1 serving	23	4	8
Italian Feast	1 serving	20	7	16
Seafood Platter	1 serving	28	7.5	39
Boiled Shrimp	1 serving	1	1.5	9
Light Fried Fish	1 serving	14	4	23
Shrimp Sampler	1 serving	23	5.5	34
Burgers/Sandwiches:				
All-American Burger	1	33	7	26
Old-Fashioned Burger	1	28	6.5	30
Chicken Fillet	1	21	6.5	25
Shoney Burger	1	36	6.5	34
Slim Jim	1	24	6.5	27
Turkey Club, Whole Wheat	1	33	8.5	56
Ham Club, Whole Wheat	1	36	8.5	92
Bacon Burger	1	40	8	35
Patty Melt	1	42	8.5	36
Charbroiled Chicken	1	17	6	44
Fish	1	13	4.5	32
Reuben	1	35	8	168
Philly Steak	1	44	9	54
Baked Ham	1	10	4	55

Shoney's

FOOD	SERVING SIZE	FAT GRAMS	CALORIE POINTS	SODIUM POINTS
Menu Items:				
Burgers/Sandwiches:				
Grilled Cheese	1	17	4	38
Grilled Bacon & Cheese	1	28	6	52
Mushroom/Swiss Burger	1	42	8.5	49
Country Fried Steak	1	26	8	65
Side Dishes:				
Baked Potato	1 (10 oz.)	0	3.5	1
Sauteed Onions	1 serving	2	0.5	10
Grecian Bread	1 serving	2	1	4
Onion Rings	1 each	3	0.5	4
Rice	1 serving	4	2	33
Sauteed Mushrooms	1 serving	7	1	42
French Fries	1 serving (3 oz.)	8	2.5	12
French Fries, Side Order	1 serving (4 oz.)	10	3.5	16
XDesserts:				
Strawberry Pie	1 piece	17	4.5	11
Hot Fudge Sundae	1	22	6	10
Strawberry Sundae	1	19	5	6
Hot Fudge Cake	1 piece	20	7	21
Apple Pie A La Mode	1 piece	23	6.5	25
Carrot Cake	1 piece	26	7	21
Walnut Brownie A La Mode	1 piece	34	8	19

TACO BELL®[1]

FOOD	SERVING SIZE	FAT GRAMS	CALORIE POINTS	SODIUM POINTS
Tacos And Tostadas:				
Taco	1	11	2.5	12
Soft Taco	1	12	3	24
Soft Taco Supreme	1	16	3.5	24
Tostada	1	11	3.5	26
Chicken Soft Taco	1	10	3	27
Taco Supreme	1	15	3	12
Burritos:				
Bean Burrito	1	14	5	50
Beef Burrito	1	21	6	57
Chicken Burrito	1	12	4.5	38
Burrito Supreme	1	22	6	51
Combo Burrito	1	16	5.5	49
Specialty Items:				
Nachos BellGrande	1 serving	35	9	43
Nachos Supreme	1 serving	27	5	20
Nachos	1 serving	18	4.5	17
Beef MexiMelt	1 serving	15	3.5	30
Chicken MexiMelt	1 serving	15	3.5	34
Mexican Pizza	1 serving	37	8	45
Pintos 'N Cheese	1 serving	9	2.5	28
Chilito	1 serving	18	5	39

Shoney's and Taco Bell

FOOD	SERVING SIZE	FAT GRAMS	CALORIE POINTS	SODIUM POINTS
Specialty Items:				
Taco Salad	1 serving	61	12	40
Taco Salad Without Shell	1 serving	31	6.5	30
Cinnamon Twists	1 serving	8	2.5	10
Side Orders And Condiments:				
Taco Sauce	1 serving	0	0	5
Hot Taco Sauce	1 serving	0	0	4
Salsa	1 serving	0	0	16
Pico De Gallo	1 serving	0	0	4
Sour Cream	1 serving	4	0.5	0
Guacamole	1 serving	2	0.5	5
Ranch Dressing	1 serving	25	3	25
Jalapeno Peppers	1 serving	0	0.5	60
Nacho Cheese Sauce	1 serving	8	1.5	17
Red Sauce	1 serving	0	0	11
Green Sauce	1 serving	0	0	6

WENDY'S[1]

FOOD	SERVING SIZE	FAT GRAMS	CALORIE POINTS	SODIUM POINTS
Sandwiches:				
Hamburger:				
Plain Single	1	15	4.5	22
Single With Everything	1	23	6	37
Big Classic	1	23	6.5	37
Junior Or Kid's Meal	1	9	3.5	26
Cheeseburger:				
Junior	1	13	4.5	33
Junior Bacon	1	25	6	38
Junior Deluxe	1	20	5.5	35
Kid's Meal	1	13	4	33
Chicken:				
Grilled	1	7	4	29
Breaded	1	20	6	32
Club	1	25	7	43
Fish	1	25	6	34
Country Fried Steak	1	26	6	38
French Fries:				
Small	1 serving	12	3	7
Medium	1 serving	17	5	10
Biggie	1 serving	22	6	12
Baked Potato:				
Plain	1 serving	0	4	1
Bacon & Cheese	1 serving	17	7	51
Broccoli & Cheese	1 serving	14	6	20
Cheese	1 serving	24	7.5	28
Chili & Cheese	1 serving	25	8	32
Sour Cream & Chives	1 serving	6	5	2
Sour Cream	1 serving	6	1	1

Taco Bell and Wendy's

FOOD	SERVING SIZE	FAT GRAMS	CALORIE POINTS	SODIUM POINTS
Chili & Accompaniments:				
Small	8 ounces	6	2.5	29
Large	12 ounces	9	4	43
Cheddar Cheese, Shredded	2 tablespoons	6	.1	5
Saltine Crackers	2 crackers	1	0.5	3
Chicken Nuggets	1 serving (6)	20	4	26
Sauces:				
Barbecue	1 packet	0	0.5	4
X Honey	1 packet	0	0.5	0
X Sweet & Sour	1 packet	0	0.5	2
X Sweet Mustard	1 packet	1	0.5	6
Garden Spot Salad Bar:				
Alfafa Sprouts	1/2 cup	0	0	0
Applesauce	2 tablespoons	0	0.5	0
Bacon Bits	2 tablespoons	2	0.5	19
Breadsticks (Small)	3	1	0.5	3
Broccoli	1/4 cup	0	0	0
Cantaloupe, Sliced	2 pieces	0	0.5	0
Carrots	1/4 cup	0	0	0
Cauliflower	1/4 cup	0	0	0
Cheddar Chips	2 tablespoons	5	1	7
Cheese, Shredded (Imitation)	2 tablespoons	4	0.5	12
Chicken Salad	2 tablespoons	5	1	6
Chives	1 tablespoon	0	0	0
Chow Mein Noodles	1/4 cup	2	0.5	2
California Cole Slaw	2 tablespoons	3	0.5	3
Cottage Cheese	2 tablespoons	1	0.5	5
Croutons	2 tablespoons	1	0.5	3
Cucumbers	2 slices	0	0	0
Eggs, Hard Cooked	2 tablespoons	3	0.5	1
Garbanzo Beans	2 tablespoons	1	0.5	0
Green Peas	2 tablespoons	0	0.5	1
Green Peppers	2 pieces	0	0	0
Honeydew Melon	2 slices	0	0.5	0
Jalapeno Peppers	1 tablespoon	0	0	7
Lettuce	1 cup	0	0	0
Mushrooms	1/4 cup	0	0	0
Olives, Black	2 tablespoons	1	0	5
Orange, Sectioned	2 pieces	0	0.5	0
Pasta Salad	2 tablespoons	4	1	5
Peaches, Sliced	1 piece	0	0.5	0
Pepperoni, Sliced	6 pieces	3	0.5	4
Pineapple, Chunked	4 pieces	0	0.5	0
Potato Salad	2 tablespoons	5	1	7
X Pudding, Chocolate	1/4 cup	3	1	3
X Pudding, Vanilla	1/4 cup	3	1	3

Wendy's

FOOD	SERVING SIZE	FAT GRAMS	CALORIE POINTS	SODIUM POINTS
Garden Spot Bar:				
Red Onions	3 rings	0	0	0
Seafood Salad	1/4 cup	4	1	13
Strawberries	4	0	0.5	0
X Strawberry Banana Dessert	1/4 cup	0	1.5	0
Sunflower Seeds And Raisins	2 tablespoons	6	1	0
Three Bean Salad	2 tablespoons	0	0.5	0
Tomato Wedges	5 pieces	0	0.5	0
Tuna Salad	2 tablespoons	6	1.5	12
Turkey Ham, Diced	2 tablespoons	1	0.5	9
Watermelon Wedges	1 piece	0	0.5	0
Salad/SuperBar:				
Salad Dressings:				
Blue Cheese	2 tablespoons	19	2.5	9
Celery Seed	2 tablespoons	11	2	5
French	2 tablespoons	10	1.5	14
X French, Sweet Red	2 tablespoons	10	2	10
Hidden Valley Ranch	2 tablespoons	10	1.5	10
Italian Caesar	2 tablespoons	16	2	11
Italian, Golden	2 tablespoons	7	1	20
Reduced Calorie:				
Bacon & Tomato	2 tablespoons	7	1	15
Italian	2 tablespoons	4	0.5	15
Salad Oil	1 tablespoon	14	1.5	0
Thousand Island	2 tablespoons	13	2	9
Wine Vinegar	1 tablespoon	0	0	0
Fresh Salads To Go/No Dressing:				
Caesar Side	1 serving	6	2	30
Deluxe Garden	1 serving	5	1.5	17
Grilled Chicken	1 serving	8	2.5	30
Side	1 serving	3	1	9
Taco	1 serving	30	8.5	42
Breadstick	1 each	3	2	11
Mexican Fiesta (SuperBar):				
Cheese Sauce	1/4 cup	2	0.5	13
Picante Sauce	1/4 cup	0	0.5	0
Refried Beans	1/4 cup	2	1	9
Rice, Spanish	1/4 cup	1	1	17
Sour Topping	2 tablespoons	4	0.5	1
Taco Chips	8 chips	6	2	1
Taco Meat	2 tablespoons	4	1	9
Taco Sauce	2 tablespoons	0	0	5
Taco Shells	1	3	0.5	2
Tortilla, Flour	1	3	1.5	9
Pasta (SuperBar):				
Alfredo Sauce	1/4 cup	1	0.5	11
Fettucini	1/2 cup	4	1.5	0
Garlic Toast	1 piece	3	1	3

Wendy's

FOOD	SERVING SIZE	FAT GRAMS	CALORIE POINTS	SODIUM POINTS
Pasta (Super Bar):				
Macaroni & Cheese	1/2 cup	6	2	14
Pasta Medley	1/2 cup	2	1	0
Red Peppers, Crushed	1 tablespoon	1	0.5	0
Romano/Parmesan Cheese, Grated	2 tablespoons	3	1	11
Rotini	1/2 cup	2	1	?-
Spaghetti Sauce	1/4 cup	0	0.5	15
Spaghetti Meat Sauce	1/4 cup	1	0.5	10
XFrosty Dairy Dessert:				
Small	12 ounces	10	4.5	9
Medium	16 ounces	13	6	11
Large	20 ounces	17	7.5	14
XChocolate Chip Cookie	1	13	4	11
XBeverages:				
Cola	16 ounces	0	1.5	0
Lemon-Lime Soft Drink	16 ounces	0	1.5	1
Lemonade	16 ounces	0	1.5	0
Hot Chocolate	6 ounces	1	1.5	5
TCBY®[1]				
XRegular Flavors	4 ounces	3	2	3
XNonfat Flavors	4 ounces	0	1.5	2
Sugar Free, Nonfat Flavors	4 ounces	0	1	2

[1]Adapted with permission from information supplied by the company.

Chapter 15

HOW DO YOU ALTER RECIPES FOR LOWER FAT CONTENT?   PLUS SAMPLE RECIPES

Our clients like to bring in their favorite recipes for help in altering them to lower the fat content. So, we thought you might like to see how to take a full fat recipe and lower the fat to more healthful levels. The recipes presented in this chapter are some of our favorites. We will show you the original recipe with the fat, calorie and sodium content. Then we will show you the lower fat version with the fat, calorie and sodium content. We used the Food Value Tables in this book to make the calculations. You can use the same technique to alter almost any of your own recipes.

GENERAL HINTS

Many recipes list a large amount of fat for use in sautéing onions, etc. or for browning meat. We find that this fat addition can be lowered substantially or cut out altogether without significantly altering the taste of the product. Spraying your pan with a non-stick spray can make it possible to leave out this fat altogether.

In one of our earlier chapters, we had a list of lower fat alternatives to try instead of the regular item such as lower fat cheeses instead of the full fat cheeses. You may want to consult this list before modifying your own recipes.

There are several ways you can lower fat in a recipe. You can leave an ingredient out. You can replace part of a high fat ingredient with a low or nonfat ingredient. You can replace all of a high fat ingredient with a low or nonfat ingredient. We will use all of these techniques in the recipes to come.

When you are baking or broiling, try spraying the food with a non stick pan spray to help keep it moist. We always bake fish on a sprayed pan and then spray the top side of the fish portion before adding herb and spice seasonings. Try an oil free marinade but remember to spray your grill.

Making or purchasing a good herb or spice blend can save time and help you turn out delicious foods. We have included two recipes for blends we have found to be quite tasty. Turn the page for the recipes.

Abbreviations used: T = tablespoon; t = teaspoon; c = cup; Chpd = chopped; oz = ounce; approx. = approximately; F = Fahrenheit; Gms = grams; Cal = Calorie; Pts = Points; lb. = pounds

SPINACH RICOTTA CHEESE TART

Original Version (8 servings)
1 prebaked pie shell
2 packages (10-oz.) frozen
    chpd spinach
1/4 c. onion, diced
1/4 c. margarine
1/4 t. ground nutmeg
Dash pepper
1 (15-oz.) carton ricotta cheese,
    part skim milk
    (approx. 2 cups)
1 c. half and half
1/2 c. grated Parmesan cheese
3 eggs, beaten slightly

Lower Fat Version (6 servings)
No pie shell
2 packages (10-oz.) frozen
    chpd spinach
1/4 c. onion, diced
1 t. margarine
1/4 t. ground nutmeg
Dash pepper
1 (15-oz.) carton ricotta cheese,
    part skim milk
    (approx. 2 cups)
1 c. skim milk
1/2 c. grated Parmesan cheese
3 eggs, beaten slightly

1. Cook spinach according to package directions.

1. Same.

2. Drain well and set aside. Sauté onion in margarine in skillet. Add spinach, nutmeg, and pepper.

2. Same.

3. Combine ricotta cheese, half and half, Parmesan cheese, and eggs in bowl, mixing thoroughly.
Stir in spinach mixture.

3. Same, except use skim milk instead of half and half.

4. Pour into prebaked pie shell and bake at 350 degrees F. for about 50 minutes or until set and lightly browned.

4. Pour into 12 inch square baking pan and bake at 350 degrees F. for about 50 minutes or until set and lightly browned.

	Whole Recipe	Per Serving	Whole Recipe	Per Serving
Fat Gms	199	25	72	12
Cal Pts	39	5	18.5	3
Sodium Pts	167	21	95	16

Note: By using fat free ricotta cheese, fat grams per serving will be lowered to 7.

MEATLOAF

Original Version (10 servings)
2 c. (4 slices) soft bread
    crumbs
1 c. chopped onion
2 eggs, beaten
2 pounds lean ground beef
    (approx. 24 oz. cooked)

2 T. Worcestershire Sauce
1 1/2 t. dry mustard
1/2 t. salt
1/2 t. freshly ground pepper
3/4 c. whole milk

Lower Fat Version (10 servings)
2 c. (4 slices) soft bread
    crumbs
1 c. chopped onion
→1 egg, plus 2 egg whites, beaten
2 pounds 7% fat ground beef with
    carrageenan (approx. 24
    oz. cooked)

2 T. Worcestershire Sauce
1 1/2 t. dry mustard
1/2 t. salt
1/2 t. freshly ground pepper
3/4 c. skim milk

1. Preheat oven to 350 degrees F.   1. Same.

2. Mix all ingredients together in a large bowl.   2. Same.

3. Grease a loaf pan.   3. Spray a loaf pan with non stick spray.

4. Press mixture into pan.   4. Same.

5. Bake for 45 minutes.   5. Same.

	Whole Recipe	Per Serving	Whole Recipe	Per Serving
Fat Gms	128	13	70	7
Cal Pts	32.5	3	25	2.5
Sodium Pts	128	13	131	13

SALMON LOAF

Original Version (8 servings)
1 can salmon, drained
1 c. (2 slices) soft bread
   crumbs
1/4 c. margarine, melted
2 eggs, beaten
1 1/2 T. onion, minced
2 t. parsley, minced
1 T. green pepper, minced
1/4 t. Worcestershire sauce
Dash of Tabasco sauce

Lower Fat Version (8 servings)
1 can salmon, drained
1 c. (2 slices) soft bread
   crumbs
Leave out margarine
1 egg, plus 2 egg whites, beaten
1 1/2 T. onion, minced
2 t. parsley, minced
1 T. green pepper, minced
1/4 t. Worcestershire sauce
Dash of Tabasco sauce

1. Preheat oven to 350 degrees F.

1. Same.

2. Grease a loaf pan.

2. Spray a loaf pan with non stick pan spray.

3. Mix all ingredients together.

3. Same.

4. Press mixture into pan.

4. Same.

5. Bake for about 35-40 minutes.

5. Same.

	Whole Recipe	Per Serving	Whole Recipe	Per Serving
Fat Gms	85	11	32	4
Cal Pts	17.5	2	11	1.5
Sodium Pts	144	18	122	15

WHITE CLAM SAUCE WITH SPAGHETTI

Original Version (4 servings)
1 (10 oz.) can minced clams
    (6 oz. clams without juice)
1 clove minced garlic
3 T. olive oil
1/4 t. thyme
1/4 t. pepper
1/4 c. parsley, chpd
1/2 c. Parmesan cheese

6 c. cooked spaghetti,
    (no oil or salt added)

1. Sauté garlic in oil.

2. Heat clams in juice from can. Add garlic, thyme and pepper.

3. Add clam mixture, parsley, and Parmesan cheese to spaghetti. Serve.

Lower Fat Version (4 servings)
1 (10 oz.) can minced clams
    (6 oz. clams without juice)
1 clove minced garlic
No oil
1/4 t. thyme
1/4 t. pepper
1/4 cup parsley, chpd
1/2 c. Parmesan cheese

6 c. cooked spaghetti,
    (no oil or salt added)

1. Simmer garlic in small amount of juice from canned clams.

2. Add clams and rest of juice to garlic. Add thyme, and pepper. Heat.

3. Same.

	Whole Recipe	Per Serving	Whole Recipe	Per Serving
Fat Gms	64	16	22	6
Cal Pts	21.5	5.5	17	4
Sodium Pts	?–	?–	?–	?–

CHILI

Original Version (4 servings)

1 pound lean ground beef

1 large onion, chpd
2 garlic cloves, chpd
3 T. olive oil
3 c. water

1 1/3 c. canned tomatoes, chpd
1 green pepper, seeded, chpd
2 T. chili powder or more
1/2 t. salt
1 t. whole cumin seed
1/2 t. ground cumin seed
1/2 t. celery seed
1/4 t. cayenne pepper
1/8 t. basil, crushed
1 small bay leaf
1 can (1 lb.) kidney beans
   (approx. 1 1/2 cups)

1. Sauté onion and garlic in oil until golden.

2. Brown ground beef in separate skillet. Drain well.

3. Transfer above ingredients to sauce pan.

4. Add rest of ingredients.

5. Simmer uncovered for 2-3 hours.

Lower Fat Version (8 servings)

1/2 pound 7% fat ground beef
   with carrageenan
1 large onion, chpd
2 garlic cloves, chpd
1 t. olive oil
3 c. water or more to taste
1 c. tomato paste, unsalted
1 (28 oz.) can tomatoes, chpd
1 green pepper, seeded, chpd
2 T. chili powder or more
1/2 t. salt
1 t. whole cumin seed
1/2 t. ground cumin seed
1/2 t. celery seed
1/4 t. cayenne pepper
1/8 t. basil, crushed
1 small bay leaf
3 cans (1 lb. each) kidney beans
   (approx. 4 1/2 cups)

1. Sauté onion and garlic in oil until golden.

2. Brown ground beef in separate skillet. Drain well.

3. Transfer above ingredients to large soup pan.

4. Add rest of ingredients.

5. Simmer uncovered for 2-3 hours.

	Whole Recipe	Per Serving	Whole Recipe	Per Serving
Fat Gms	99	25	31	4
Cal Pts	23.5	6	25	3
Sodium Pts	143	36	299	37

Note: The Lower Fat Version makes twice as many servings as the Original Version.

SOUR CREAM MUFFINS

Original Version (12 muffins)
1 egg, beaten
1 c. sour cream
2 T. melted margarine
2 c. sifted all-purpose flour
1/4 c. sugar
2 t. baking powder
1/2 t. baking soda
1/2 t. salt
1/4 c. whole milk

Lower Fat Version (12 muffins)
1 egg, beaten
1 c. plain nonfat yogurt
2 T. melted margarine
2 c. sifted all-purpose flour
1/4 c. sugar
2 t. baking powder
1/2 t. baking soda
1/2 t. salt
1/4 c. skim milk

1. Preheat oven to 400 degrees F.

1. Same.

2. Beat egg and sour cream until light.

2. Beat egg and yogurt together.

3. Add rest of ingredients. Stir only until dry ingredients are moistened. Do not overmix.

3. Same.

4. Fill twelve 2 3/4" muffin cups half full with the batter. Bake in oven about 20 minutes.

4. Same.

	Whole Recipe	Per Serving	Whole Recipe	Per Serving
Fat Gms	75	6	33	3
Cal Pts	23	2	20	1.5
Sodium Pts	119	10	119	10

SOUR CREAM CORN BREAD

Original Version (8 servings)
3/4 c. yellow corn meal
1 c. unsifted all-purpose flour
1/4 c. sugar
2 t. baking powder
1/2 t. baking soda
1/2 t. salt
1 c. sour cream
1/4 c. whole milk
1 egg, beaten
2 T. vegetable oil

Lower Fat Version (8 servings)
3/4 c. yellow corn meal
1 c. unsifted all-purpose flour
1/4 c. sugar
2 t. baking powder
1/2 t. baking soda
1/2 t. salt
1 c. plain nonfat yogurt
1/4 c. skim milk
1 egg, beaten
2 T. vegetable oil

SOUR CREAM CORN BREAD (continued)

1. Preheat oven to 425 degrees.	1. Same.
2. Stir all ingredients together just enough to blend. Do not overmix.	2. Same.
3. Pour into 8" square greased pan and bake about 20 minutes.	3. Spray an 8" square pan with non stick pan spray. Pour into pan and bake about 20 minutes.

	Whole Recipe	Per Serving	Whole Recipe	Per Serving
Fat Gms	60	8	38	5
Cal Pts	19	2.5	18.5	2.5
Sodium Pts	102	13	107	14

VEGETABLE AND OLIVE SALAD

Original Version (Serves 6)

1 head of butterhead lettuce, torn

1 head of romaine lettuce, torn
36 pitted ripe olives
1 c. radishes, sliced
2 carrots, grated
1 c. celery, sliced
1 c. plain nonfat yogurt
1 T. Dijon mustard
1/4 t. salt
1/4 t. pepper

Lower Fat Version (Serves 6)

1 head of butterhead lettuce, torn

1 head of romaine lettuce, torn
18 pitted ripe olives
1 c. radishes, sliced
2 carrots, grated
1 c. celery, sliced
1 c. plain nonfat yogurt
1 T. Dijon mustard
1/4 t. salt
1/4 t. pepper

1. Mix lettuces, olives, radishes, carrots, and celery together in large bowl.	1. Same.
2. Combine yogurt, mustard, salt, and pepper. Add to greens and toss well.	2. Same.

	Whole Recipe	Per Serving	Whole Recipe	Per Serving
Fat Gms	18	3	9	2
Cal Pts	5	1	4	0.5
Sodium Pts	110	18	80	13

PRETZEL OVEN-FRIED CHICKEN

Original Version (6 servings)
6 chicken breast halves

1 c. sour cream
1 T. lemon juice
1 t. Worcestershire sauce
1/2 t. salt
1/4 t. pepper
4 oz. crushed pretzels

1. Preheat oven to 350 degrees F.

2. Mix sour cream, lemon juice,
    Worcestershire sauce, salt,
    and pepper.

3. Dip the chicken pieces in the
    mixture and coat well.

4. Roll them in the crushed pretzels.

5. Place the chicken pieces in a
    greased pan and bake for about
    50 minutes or until crisp and brown.

Lower Fat Version (6 servings)
3 whole chicken breasts,
    boneless, skinless, halved
1 c. plain nonfat yogurt
1 T. lemon juice
1 t. Worcestershire sauce
1/2 t. salt
1/4 t. pepper
4 oz. crushed pretzels

1. Same.

2. Mix yogurt, lemon juice,
    Worcestershire sauce, salt,
    and pepper.

3. Same.

4. Same.

5. Place the chicken pieces in
    a pan sprayed with non stick
    pan spray. Rest same.

	Whole Recipe	Per Serving	Whole Recipe	Per Serving
Fat Gms	92	15	22	4
Cal Pts	25	4	19.5	3
Sodium Pts	159	27	159	27

CHICKEN STROGANOFF

Original Version (4 servings)
1 medium onion, chpd
1/4 c. olive oil
1/2 lb. mushrooms, sliced
1 T. flour
2 t. paprika
1/4 t. salt
1/4 t. basil
1/4 t. thyme
1/2 c. chicken broth
1/2 c. dry vermouth
1/2 c. sour cream
2 c. cooked chicken, diced
2 t. lemon juice
1 t. dill weed

Lower Fat Version (4 servings)
1 medium onion, chpd
1 t. olive oil
1/2 lb. mushrooms, sliced
1 T. flour
2 t. paprika
1/4 t. salt
1/4 t. basil
1/4 t. thyme
1/2 c. chicken broth
1/2 c. dry vermouth
1/2 c. nonfat plain yogurt
2 c. cooked chicken, diced
2 t. lemon juice
1 t. dill weed

1. Sauté onion in oil until golden.

1. Same.

2. Add mushrooms. Cook and stir 3 to 5 minutes longer. Blend in flour, paprika, salt, basil, and thyme. Cook 1 minute. Remove from heat.

2. Same.

3. Stir in chicken broth and wine. Return to heat. Cook, stirring constantly until mixture thickens. Cover. Simmer 5 minutes.

3. Same.

4. Remove from heat. Blend in sour cream, chicken, lemon juice, and dill. Heat thoroughly, but do not allow to boil.

4. Remove from heat. Blend in yogurt, chicken, lemon juice, and dill. Heat thoroughly, but do not allow to boil.

5. Serve over hot cooked noodles. (Not included in calculations below.)

5. Same.

	Whole Recipe	Per Serving	Whole Recipe	Per Serving
Fat Gms	88	22	17	4
Cal Pts	19.5	5	13	3
Sodium Pts	66	17	66	17

ROAST PORK

We are presenting only one version here because this recipe contains no ingredients, except the pork, which contains fat. (10 servings)

2 1/2 pounds pork loin strip, trimmed of all visible fat
1 green onion, chpd
1 clove garlic, chpd
1 T. picante sauce
2 T. sherry
2 T. soy sauce
1 t. brown sugar
1/4 t. salt
1/4 t. paprika

1. Place pork in a glass pan. Mix rest of ingredients and coat pork with the mixture. Leave overnight in the refrigerator. Turn over once or twice.

2. Remove from marinade. Roast in preheated oven for 40 minutes per pound. Baste with marinade during baking.

3. Remove from oven. Cool and slice thin. Serve at room temperature.

	Whole Recipe	Per Serving
Fat Gms	105	11
Cal Pts	30	3
Sodium Pts	151	15

BAKED ORANGE ROUGHY

Original Version (4 servings)
1 pound orange roughy
2 T. olive oil
Garlic powder
Onion powder
Paprika
Dill weed
Salt
Pepper

Lower Fat Version (4 servings)
1 pound orange roughy
Pan spray
Garlic powder
Onion powder
Paprika
Dill weed
Salt
Pepper

1. Preheat oven to 400 degrees F.
2. Coat fish with oil.

3. Sprinkle rest of ingredients to taste on fish.

1. Same.
2. Spray pan and fish with non stick pan spray.
3. Same.

BAKED ORANGE ROUGHY (continued)

4. Bake for approx. 15 minutes   4. Same.
   in oven.

	Whole Recipe	Per Serving	Whole Recipe	Per Serving
Fat Gms	32	8	4	1
Cal Pts	7	2	4	1
Sodium Pts	12	3	12	3

SOUR CREAM POTATO SALAD

Original Version (6 servings)
6 c. cooked potatoes, diced
1/4 c. onion, chpd
1/4 c. celery, chpd
1/2 c. parsley, minced
1 t. celery seed
1/2 t. salt
1/2 t. pepper
4 eggs, hard boiled
1 c. sour cream
1/2 c. mayonnaise

1/4 c. vinegar
1 t. prepared mustard
3/4 c. pared cucumber, diced

Lower Fat Version (6 servings)
6 c. cooked potatoes, diced
1/4 c. onion, chpd
1/4 c. celery, chpd
1/2 c. parsley, minced
1 t. celery seed
1/2 t. salt
1/2 t. pepper
2 eggs, hard boiled
1 c. plain nonfat yogurt
1/2 c. fat free salad dressing,
   mayonnaise type
1/4 c. vinegar
1 t. prepared mustard
3/4 c. cucumber, diced

1. Mix potatoes, onion, celery,   1. Same.
   parsley, celery seed, salt,
   pepper, and eggs in large
   bowl.

2. Combine sour cream, mayon-   2. Combine yogurt, fat free salad
   naise, vinegar, and mustard.   dressing, vinegar, and mustard.

3. Pour over potato mixture and   3. Same.
   mix well. Add cucumber
   just before serving.

	Whole Recipe	Per Serving	Whole Recipe	Per Serving
Fat Gms	148	25	10	2
Cal Pts	29.5	5	17	3
Sodium Pts	98	16	76	13

ZUCCHINI IN FOIL

Original Version (4 servings)
4 medium zucchini squash
1/4 cup olive oil
Garlic powder
Dill weed
Herb blend

1. Place zucchini on squares of aluminum foil. Add 1 T. oil to each squash. Sprinkle to taste with other ingredients.

2. Wrap foil around squash and grill over a hot grill for approx. 30 minutes.

Lower Fat Version (4 servings)
4 medium zucchini squash
Pan spray
Garlic powder
Dill weed
Herb blend

1. Place zucchini on squares of aluminum foil. Spray each squash with non stick pan spray. Sprinkle to taste with other ingredients.

2. Same.

	Whole Recipe	Per Serving	Whole Recipe	Per Serving
Fat Gms	56	14	0	0
Cal Pts	8	2	2	0.5
Sodium Pts	0	0	0	0

SPICE BLENDS (ALSO SALT FREE)

CAJUN SPICE BLEND
(Makes about 1/2 cup)
1/4 cup paprika
1 T. ground hot red pepper
1 T. ground white pepper
1 T. ground black pepper
1 T. onion powder
1 T. garlic powder
2 t. oregano
1 t. thyme

CURRY BLEND
(Makes about 1/2 cup)
1 T. turmeric
1 T. coriander
1 T. cumin
1 T. garlic powder
1 T. ground ginger
1 T. ground cardamom seed
1 t. celery seed
1 t, ground black pepper
1 t. mustard powder
1 t. red pepper
1 t. ground ginger

Note: Fat, calorie, and sodium free.

SALMON DIP

Original Version (16 servings–approx. 1/4 c.)

1 (1 lb.) can salmon
1 (8 oz.) pkg. cream cheese
1 T. lemon juice
1 t. prepared horseradish
1/2 c. pecans, chpd
3 T. parsley, minced
2 t. onion, minced

1. Drain salmon, break up

2. Combine all ingredients. Mix thoroughly.

3. Chill for several hours before serving.

4. Serve with assorted crackers.

Lower Fat Version (16 servings–approx. 1/4 c.)

1 (1 lb.) can salmon
1 (8 oz.) pkg. fat free cream cheese
1 T. lemon juice
1 t. prepared horseradish
1/4 c. pecans, chpd
3 T. parsley, minced
2 t. onion, minced

1. Same.

2. Same.

3. Same.

4. Same.

	Whole Recipe	Per Serving	Whole Recipe	Per Serving
Fat Gms	124	8	35	2
Cal Pts	21.5	1.5	12.5	1
Sodium Pts	132	8	156	10

MY FAVORITE FOODS NOT LISTED/NOTES

APPENDIX A
METROPOLITAN HEIGHT/WEIGHT TABLES

The Metropolitan Life Foundation provided these guidelines in 1959 and 1983. Weights in the 1983 version were based on the lowest death rates for men and women at ages 25 to 59 for various heights and body frame sizes.

The first table below assists you in determining your frame size and the second table is the 1983 Metropolitan Height and Weight table.

Both tables are provided courtesy of the Metropolitan Life Insurance Company.

TO MAKE AN APPROXIMATION OF YOUR FRAME SIZE. . .

Extend your arm and bend the forearm upward at a 90 degree angle. Keep fingers straight and turn the inside of your wrist toward your body. If you have a caliper, use it to measure the space between the two prominent bones on **either** side of your elbows. Without a caliper, place thumb and index finger of your other hand on these two bones. Measure the space between your fingers against a ruler or tape measure. Compare it with these tables that list elbow measurements for **medium-framed** men and women. Measurements lower than those listed indicate you have a small frame. Higher measurements indicate a large frame.

Height in 1" Heels MEN	Elbow Breadth	Height in 1" Heels WOMEN	Elbow Breadth
5'2"—5'3"	2 1/2"—2 7/8"	4'10"—4'11"	2 1/4"—2 1/2"
5'4"—5'7"	2 5/8"—2 7/8"	5'0"—5'3"	2 1/4"—2 1/2"
5'8"—5'11"	2 3/4"—3"	5'4"—5'7"	2 3/8"—2 5/8"
6'0"—6'3"	2 3/4"—3 1/8"	5'8"—5'11"	2 3/8"—2 5/8"
6'4"	2 7/8"—3 1/4"	6'0"	2 1/2"—2 3/4"

1983 METROPOLITAN HEIGHT AND WEIGHT TABLES

The weights on the tables are representative of adults (between the ages of 25-59), based on lowest mortality (death rates). The weight is in pounds according to frame size in indoor clothing weighing 5 pounds for men and 3 pounds for women; height includes shoes with 1" heels.

Height Inches	MEN Small Frame	MEN Medium Frame	MEN Large Frame	WOMEN Small Frame	WOMEN Medium Frame	WOMEN Large Frame
58				102–111	109–121	118–131
59				103–113	111–123	120–134
60				104–115	113–126	122–137
61				106–118	115–129	125–140
62	128–134	131–141	138–150	108–121	118–132	128–143
63	130–136	133–143	140–153	111–124	121–135	131–147
64	132–138	135–145	142–156	114–127	124–138	134–151
65	134–140	137–148	144–160	117–130	127–141	137–155
66	136–142	139–151	146–164	120–133	130–144	140–159
67	138–145	142–154	149–168	123–136	133–147	143–163
68	140–148	145–157	152–172	126–139	136–150	146–167
69	142–151	148–160	155–176	129–142	139–153	149–170
70	144–154	151–163	158–180	132–145	142–156	152–173
71	146–157	154–166	161–184	135–148	145–159	155–176
72	149–160	157–170	164–188	138–151	148–162	158–179
73	152–164	160–174	168–192			
74	155–168	164–178	172–197			
75	158–172	167–182	176–202			
76	162–176	171–187	181–207			

APPENDIX B

TABLE OF TOTAL FIBER AND SOLUBLE FIBER IN PLANT FOODS

The following fiber information was adapted with permission from : James W. Anderson, M.D., **PLANT FIBER IN FOODS,** Second Edition, HCF Nutrition Research Foundation, Inc., P.O. Box 22124, Lexington, KY 40522, 1990.

HOW DO I FIGURE MY DAILY LEVELS OF TOTAL FIBER AND SOLUBLE FIBER?

The recommended daily fiber goals are to consume 20-30 grams of total fiber per each 1000 calories. Include at least 13-20 grams of soluble fiber per day for helping lowering blood levels of cholesterol, triglycerides, and glucose (sugar).

Check the chart below to determine your total daily fiber needs based on your estimated daily calorie needs. For simplicity, we have converted total fiber grams into total fiber points and have rounded soluble fiber grams to the nearest gram. **One total fiber point is equal to 2 grams of total fiber.**

For example, you can use the chart on page 27 in Chapter Seven to estimate that you need to eat 2000 calories per day. Notice on the chart below that this means you need to eat foods which will provide 20 Total Fiber Points and at least 13-20 grams of soluble fiber.

DAILY LEVELS OF TOTAL FIBER AND SOLUBLE FIBER

CALORIES PER DAY	TOTAL FIBER GRAMS	TOTAL FIBER POINTS	GRAMS SOLUBLE FIBER
1400	28	14	13-20
1500	30	15	13-20
1600	32	16	13-20
1700	34	17	13-20
1800	36	18	13-20
1900	38	19	13-20
2000	40	20	13-20
2100	42	21	13-20
2200	44	22	13-20
2300	46	23	13-20
2400	48	24	13-20
2500	50	25	13-20

FOOD	SERVING SIZE	TOTAL FIBER POINTS	GRAMS SOLUBLE FIBER
BREADS, CEREALS AND GRAINS			
Bread:			
Bagel, Plain	1/2	0.5	trace
Biscuit, Baked	1	0.5	trace
Bran	1 slice	1	trace
Cellulose	2 slices	2.5	1
Corn Bread	1 1/2" cube	0.5	trace
Cracked Wheat	1 slice	1	trace
French	1 slice	0.5	trace
Mixed Grain	1 slice	1	trace
Mixed Grain "Lite"	1 slice	3	trace
Oatmeal	1 slice	1	1
Pumpernickel	1 slice	1.5	1
Raisin	1 slice	0.5	trace
Rye	1 slice	1	1
Rye (German)	1 slice	1	trace
Wheat Or White "Lite"	2 slices	3	trace
White, Enriched	1 slice	0.5	trace
100% Whole Wheat	1 slice	1	trace
Crackers:			
Graham	3 (2 1/2" square)	trace	trace
Oat Bran Graham, HV*	3 (2 1/2" square)	0.5	trace
Saltines	6	0.5	trace
Whole Wheat, Snack	5	1	trace
Taco Shell	2	0.5	trace
Tortilla, Corn	1	0.5	trace
Barley, Pearled	2 tablespoons	1.5	1
Flour:			
All-Purpose	2 1/2 tablespoons	0.5	trace
Buck Wheat	2 1/2 tablespoons	0.5	trace
Oat	5 tablespoons	2	2
Rye	2 1/2 tablespoons	0.5	1
Whole Wheat	2 1/2 tablespoons	1	trace
Macaroni, Cooked:			
White	1/2 cup	0.5	trace
Whole Wheat	1/2 cup	1	trace
Noodles, Cooked:			
Egg	1/2 cup	0.5	trace
Spinach	1/2 cup	0.5	1
Popcorn, Popped	3 cups	1	trace
Rice, White Or Wild, Cooked	2/3 cup	0.5	trace

*HV = Health Valley

FOOD	SERVING SIZE	TOTAL FIBER POINTS	GRAMS SOLUBLE FIBER
Spaghetti, Cooked:			
White	1/2 cup	0.5	trace
Whole Wheat	1/2 cup	1.5	1
Cereal:			
All Bran, Kellogg's	1/3 cup	4.5	1
All Bran, With Extra Fiber, Kellogg's	1/2 cup	7	1
Benefit	3/4 cup	2.5	3
Cheerios	1 1/4 cups	1.5	1
Corn Bran, Uncooked	1/3 cup	10	trace
Cornmeal	2 1/2 tablespoons	trace	trace
Corn Flakes, Kellogg's	1 cup	0.5	trace
Cream of Wheat, Regular, Dry	2 1/2 tablespoons	0.5	trace
Crispy Oats, Kolin	1/2 cup	1	1
Fiber One	1/2 cup	6	1
40% Bran Flakes	2/3 cup	2	trace
Fruit And Fitness, HV*	1/3 cup	1.5	1
Grapenuts	1/4 cup	1.5	1
Grits, Corn, Quick, Dry	3 tablespoons	0.5	trace
Heartwise	1 cup	3	3
Just Right, Fiber Nuggets	2/3 cup	0.5	trace
Nutri-Grain, Wheat	2/3 cup	1.5	1
Oat Bran, Dry	2/3 cup	4	4
Oat Bran, Cold Cereal, Quakers	3/4 cup	1.5	2
Oat Bran Crunch, Kolin	1/2 cup	2.5	3
Oat Bran Flakes, HV*	1/2 cup	1	1
Oat Bran Cereal, Apples & Cinnamon, Dry, HV*	1/4 cup	1.5	1
Oat Bran O's, HV*	3/4 cup	1	1
Oatflakes	1 1/3 cups	2	2
Oatbran And Oatgerm	1/3 cup	2	2
Oatmeal, Dry	1/3 cup	1.5	1
Product 19	1 cup	0.5	trace
Puffed Rice	1 cup	trace	trace
Puffed Wheat	1 cup	0.5	1
Quaker Oat Squares	1/2 cup	1	1
Raisin Bran	3/4 cup	2.5	1
Real Oat Bran Cereal Almond Crunch, HV*	1/2 cup	2	2
Rice Krispies	1 cup	trace	trace
Shredded Wheat	2/3 cup	2	1

*HV = Health Valley

FOOD	SERVING SIZE	TOTAL FIBER POINTS	GRAMS SOLUBLE FIBER
Shredded Wheat & Bran	2/3 cup	1.5	1
Special K	1 cup	0.5	trace
Total, Whole Wheat	1 cup	1.5	1
Wheat Flakes	3/4 cup	1	trace
Wheaties	2/3 cup	1	1
Wheat Bran	1 cup	12.5	2
Wheat Germ	3 tablespoons	2	1

FRUITS

FOOD	SERVING SIZE	TOTAL FIBER POINTS	GRAMS SOLUBLE FIBER
Apple:			
Raw, Without Skin	1 small	1	1
Raw, With Skin	2 small	3	2
Applesauce, Canned, Unsweetened	1/2 cup	1	1
Apricots:			
Canned, Drained	4 halves	0.5	1
Dried	7 halves	1	1
Raw, With Skin	4 fruits	2	2
Avocado	1/4	1	1
Banana, Raw	1 small	1	1
Blackberries, Raw	3/4 cup	2	1
Blueberries, Raw	3/4 cup	0.5	trace
Cantaloupe	1 cup cubed	0.5	trace
Cherries:			
Black, Raw	12 large	0.5	1
Red, Canned	1/2 cup	1	1
Cranberries, Raw	1/2 cup	1	1
Currants, Black, Raw	1 cup	2	2
Dates, Dried	5 medium	1	1
Figs, Dried	3 medium	2.5	2
Fruit Cocktail, Canned	1/2 cup	1	1
Gooseberries, Raw	1 1/2 cups	3	2
Grapefruit:			
Canned, Unsweetened	1/2 cup	0.5	1
Raw	1/2 medium	1	1
Grapes:			
Red, Raw	15 small	trace	trace
White, Raw	15 small	0.5	trace
Guava, Raw	1 1/3 fruit	3	1
Kiwi, Raw	1 large	1	1
Loganberries, Canned	3/4 cup	2	1
Lychees, Canned	10	0.5	1
Mango, Raw	1/2 small	1.5	2

FOOD	SERVING SIZE	TOTAL FIBER POINTS	GRAMS SOLUBLE FIBER
Honeydew Melon	1 cup	0.5	trace
Nectarine, Raw	1	1	1
Orange:			
Mandarin, Canned	3/4 cup	0.5	trace
Raw	1 small`	1.5	2
Passion Fruit, Raw	3 fruits	trace	trace
Peach:			
Canned, Water Pack	1/2 cup	1	1
Dried	1/3 cup	0.5	1
Raw	2 medium	2	2
Pear:			
Canned	1/2 cup	2	1
Raw, With Skin	1/2 large	1.5	1
Pineapple:			
Canned	1/3 cup	0.5	trace
Raw	3/4 cup	0.5	trace
Plums:			
Canned	1/2 cup	1.5	1
Red, Raw	2 medium	1	1
Pomegranate, Raw	1/2	1.5	1
Prunes:			
Dried	6 medium	1.5	2
Dried, Cooked	1/2 cup	1.5	2
Raisins	1/2 cup	1	1
Raspberries:			
Canned	1/2 cup	2	1
Red, Raw	1 cup	1.5	1
Rhubarb, Raw	2 cups	2	2
Strawberries, Raw	1 1/4 cups	1.5	1
Watermelon, Raw	1 1/4 cups	0.5	trace

NUTS

FOOD	SERVING SIZE	TOTAL FIBER POINTS	GRAMS SOLUBLE FIBER
Almonds	6 nuts	0.5	trace
Peanuts, Roasted	10 large	0.5	trace
Peanut Butter, Smooth	3 tablespoons	1.5	1
Sesame Or Sunflower Seeds	1 tablespoon	0.5	trace
Walnuts, English	4 whole	0.5	trace

VEGETABLES

FOOD	SERVING SIZE	TOTAL FIBER POINTS	GRAMS SOLUBLE FIBER
Asparagus:			
Canned	1/2 cup	1.5	1
Cooked	1/2 cup	1	1

FOOD	SERVING SIZE	TOTAL FIBER POINTS	GRAMS SOLUBLE FIBER
Beans:			
Black, Cooked	1/2 cup	3	2
Broad, Cooked	1 cup	5	2
Butter, Cooked	1/2 cup	3.5	3
Garbanzo, Canned	1 cup	4	1
Green:			
Canned/Frozen, Cooked	1/2 cup	1	1
French, Cooked	1/2 cup	1.5	1
Kidney:			
Canned	1 cup	8	4
Dried, Cooked	1/2 cup	3.5	3
Lentils, Dried, Cooked	1/2 cup	2.5	1
Lima, Canned	1/2 cup	2	1
Mung, Dried, Cooked	1/2 cup	1.5	1
Navy, Dried, Cooked	1/2 cup	3.5	2
Pinto:			
Canned	1/2 cup	3	1
Dried, Cooked	1/2 cup	3	2
Pork & Beans, Canned	1/2 cup	2.5	3
Soy, Dried, Uncooked	1/3 cup	5.5	4
White, Great Northern:			
Canned	1/2 cup	3.5	2
Dried, Cooked	1/2 cup	2.5	1
Sprouts, Raw	1 cup	1	1
Beets, Canned Or Fresh, Cooked	1/2 cup	1	1
Broccoli, Cooked	1/2 cup	1	1
Brussels Sprouts, Cooked	1 cup	4	4
Cabbage:			
Red, Cooked	1/2 cup	1.5	1
Red Or Savoy, Raw	1 cup	1.5	1
Savoy, Cooked	1/2 cup	1	1
White, Raw	1 cup	1	1
Carrots:			
Canned Or Cooked	1/2 cup	1	1
Raw	1 (7 1/2" long)	1	1
Cauliflower:			
Cooked	1/2 cup	0.5	trace
Raw	1 cup	1	1
Celeriac	1/2 cup	1.5	2
Celery, Raw	1 cup, chopped	1	1

FOOD	SERVING SIZE	TOTAL FIBER POINTS	GRAMS SOLUBLE FIBER
Corn:			
Canned, Whole Kernel	1/2 cup	1	trace
On Cob, Cooked	1 ear (6" long)	1	trace
Cucumber, Raw	1 cup	0.5	trace
Eggplant, Cooked	1/2 cup	0.5	trace
Endive	1 cup	0.5	1
Kale, Chopped, Frozen	1/2 cup	1.5	1
Leeks, Cooked	1/2 cup	0.5	1
Lettuce:			
Butterhead	1 cup	trace	trace
Iceberg	1 cup	0.5	trace
Mushrooms, Raw	1 cup	0.5	trace
Okra, Frozen, Cooked	1 cup	4	2
Olives, Canned	10 small	0.5	trace
Onion, Cooked Or Raw	1/2 cup chopped	1	1
Parsnips, Cooked	1/2 cup	1.5	2
Peas:			
Blackeye, Canned	1/2 cup	2.5	1
Chick, Dried, Cooked	1/2 cup	2	1
Green:			
Canned	1/2 cup	1.5	trace
Fresh, Cooked	1/2 cup	1	1
Frozen, Cooked	1/2 cup	2	1
Snow, Cooked	1/2 cup	0.5	1
Split, Dried, Cooked	1/2 cup	1.5	1
Pepper, Green, Raw	1 cup chopped	1	1
Potato:			
White, Fresh, With Skin	1/2 cup	1	1
Sweet, Canned	1/3 cup	0.5	trace
Sweet, Cooked	1/3 cup	1.5	1
Pumpkin, Fresh, Cooked	1 cup	0.5	trace
Radishes	1 cup slices	0.5	1
Spinach, Cooked	1/2 cup	1	1
Squash:			
Yellow, Crookneck, Frozen	1/2 cup	0.5	trace
Zucchini, Cooked	1/2 cup	0.5	1
Zucchini, Raw	1 cup	1	1
Tomatoes:			
Canned	1/2 cup	0.5	1
Raw	1 medium	0.5	trace
Sauce	1/3 cup	0.5	1
Turnips, Cooked	1/2 cup	2.5	2

FOOD	SERVING SIZE	TOTAL FIBER POINTS	GRAMS SOLUBLE FIBER
Vegetable Juice, Canned	1/2 cup	0.5	trace
Yams, Cooked	1/3 cup	0.5	trace

MISCELLANEOUS

FOOD	SERVING SIZE	TOTAL FIBER POINTS	GRAMS SOLUBLE FIBER
Angel Food Cake	1/12 cake	0.5	trace
Blueberry Muffin, Commercial	1	0.5	trace
Bran Muffin, Commercial	1	0.5	trace
Gingersnaps	3	trace	trace
Oat Bran Animal Cookies, HV*	6	1	1
Oat Bran Fancy Fruit Muffins, HV*	1	1.5	2
Oat Bran Fruit Jumbo Cookies, HV*	1	0.5	trace
Oat Bran Fruit & Nut Cookies, HV*	2	1	1
Oat Bran Jumbo Fruit Bar, HV*	1	1	1
Oat Bran Muffin, Commercial	1	0.5	trace

CONCENTRATED FIBERS

FOOD	SERVING SIZE	TOTAL FIBER POINTS	GRAMS SOLUBLE FIBER
Citrucel	1 tablespoon	1	2
Citrus Pectin	1 tablespoon	3	6
Fibrim	1 teaspoon	0.5	1
Metamucil	1 teaspoon	1.5	2
Metamucil, Sugar Free	1 teaspoon	1.5	3

*HV = Health Valley

APPENDIX C
SUGGESTED READINGS

LIVING WITHOUT DIETING, 1992, soft cover, By John P. Foreyt, Ph.D., and G. Ken Goodrick, Ph.D.

FAT IS NOT A FOUR-LETTER WORD, 1992, soft cover, By Charles Roy Schroeder, Ph.D.

THE NEW FITNESS FORMULA OF THE 90'S: A Compilation of 12 Points of View, Written by the Nation's Top Health Writers and Fitness Authorities, 1990, soft cover

THE NEW FIT OR FAT, 1991, soft cover, By Covert Bailey

THE EXERCISE HABIT: Your Personal Road Map to Developing a Lifelong Exercise Commitment, 1992, By James Gavin

THE LIVING HEART BRAND NAME SHOPPER'S GUIDE, 1992, soft cover with spiral binding, By Michael DeBakey, Antonio M. Gotto, Jr., Lynne W. Scott, and John P. Foreyt, Ph.D.

EATING ON THE RUN, 1992, soft cover, By Evelyn Tribole, M.S., R.D.

THE TUFTS GUIDE TO TOTAL NUTRITION, 1990, soft cover, By Stanley Gershoff, Ph.D., with Catherine Whitney

JANE BRODY'S NUTRITION BOOK, 1987, soft cover, By Jane Brody

QUICK & HEALTHY: For People Who Say They Don't Have Time to Cook Healthy Meals, 1991, By Brenda J. Ponichtera, R.D.

MEXICAN LIGHT COOKING: Easy, Healthy, Low-Calorie Recipes from Nachos to Tacos, 1992, hard cover, spiral bound, By Kathi Long

ITALIAN LIGHT COOKING: Easy, Healthy, Low-Calorie Recipes from Pizza to Pesto, 1992, hard cover, spiral bound, By Marie Simmons

COOKING A' LA HEART, 1992, soft cover, By Linda Hachfeld, M.P.H., R.D. and Betsy Eklyn, M.S.

A TOUCH OF DIABETES: A Guide for People Who Have Type II Non-Insulin-Dependent Diabetes, 1991, soft cover, By Lois Jovanovic-Peterson, M.D., Charles M. Peterson, M.D., and Morton B. Stone

THE UCSD HEALTHY DIET FOR DIABETES: A Comprehensive Nutritional Guide and Cookbook, 1990, soft cover, By Susan Algert, M.S., R.D., Barbara Grasse, R.D., C.D.E., and Annie Durning, M.S., R.D.

LEARNING TO LIVE WELL WITH DIABETES, 1991, soft cover, Edited by Donnell D. Etzwiler, M.D., Marion J. Franz, R.D., M.S., Priscilla Hollander, M.D., and Judy Ostro Joynes, R.N., M.A.

WALKING: A Complete Guide to the Complete Exercise, 1992, soft cover, By Casey Meyers

ABOUT THE AUTHORS

Patricia M. Stein, M.S., M.A., is a Registered and Licensed Dietitian in private practice in the Kansas City area. She is also the owner of a mail order catalog company featuring books on nutrition, exercise and eating disorders. She was formerly Assistant Professor of Clinical Dietetics and Clinical Dietitian, University of Kansas Medical Center. Her specialties are helping people set up weight management programs and working with people who have compulsive eating habits. She and Barbara Unell are the authors of the book, *ANOREXIA NERVOSA: Find The Lifeline*, Compcare Publications.

Norma Winn, M.S., is a Registered and Licensed Dietitian and Internship Director and Associate Professor of Clinical Dietetics at the University of Kansas Medical Center. She has worked with people receiving gastric bypass operations from the Morbid Obesity Clinic at K.U. She is an authority on the nutrition treatment of surgery and burn patients.

Stein and Winn have co-authored several publications, including the compilation and editing of three editions of *THE KANSAS DIET MANUAL*, 1972, 1977, 1981. Norma Winn is co-editor along with Barbara Amick, R.D. of the 1987 edition of *THE KANSAS DIET MANUAL*.

ACKNOWLEDGMENTS

We wish to express appreciation to Virginia Toews Stucky, R.D., M.S. for developing the "point" concept. Thanks also to Barbara Amick, R.D., and Gayle Lopes, R.D. for sharing information from the 1992 edition of *THE KANSAS DIET MANUAL*.

ORDER FORM

Item No.	Item	Price/ Each	Quantity	Total
1008A	THE "CAN HAVE" DIET AND MORE	$7.50		
1008A	For orders of 20 or more copies of THE "CAN HAVE" DIET AND MORE!, deduct 40% off the $7.50 price	$4.50		
TOTAL PRICE OF BOOKS				
POSTAGE AND HANDLING CHARGES: For orders under $30.00, add $3.00 to total price of books. For orders over $30.00, add 10% of total cost of books.				
SALES TAX: Kansas residents, add 6.5% to total price of books and the postage and handling charges.				
TOTAL: Include price of books, tax (KS residents only), and postage and handling.				

☐ Yes, please send me a free NCES catalog.

To receive your books, please enclose your check or money order made out to: NCES.

Mail to:
NCES
1904 East 123rd Street
Olathe, KS 66061

Your Mailing Address:
Name _____
Address _____
City _____ State _____ Zip _____
Telephone _____
            Area Code   Number